Leading Antenatal Classes
A practical guide

To all parents – past, present and future

Commissioning editor: Mary Seager
Desk editor: Deena Burgess
Production controller: Chris Jarvis
Development editor: Caroline Savage
Cover design: Greg Harris

Leading Antenatal Classes

A practical guide

Second edition

Judith Schott and Judy Priest

Illustrations by Helen Chown

OXFORD AUCKLAND BOSTON JOHANNESBURG MELBOURNE NEW DELHI

Books for Midwives
An imprint of Butterworth-Heinemann
Linacre House, Jordan Hill, Oxford OX2 8DP
225 Wildwood Avenue, Woburn, MA 01801-2041
A division of Reed Educational and Professional Publishing Ltd

A member of the Reed Elsevier plc group

First published 1991
Reprinted 1991, 1993, 1994, 1996, 1997, 1998, 1999, 2001
Second edition 2002

British Library Cataloguing in Publication Data
Schott, Judith
Leading antenatal classes. – 2nd ed.
I. Title II. Priest, Judy
618.2′4

ISBN 0 7506 4984 4

For information on all Butterworth-Heinemann publications visit our website at www.bh.com

Typeset by David Gregson Associates, Beccles, Suffolk
Printed and bound in Great Britain by Biddles Ltd, Guildford and Kings Lynn

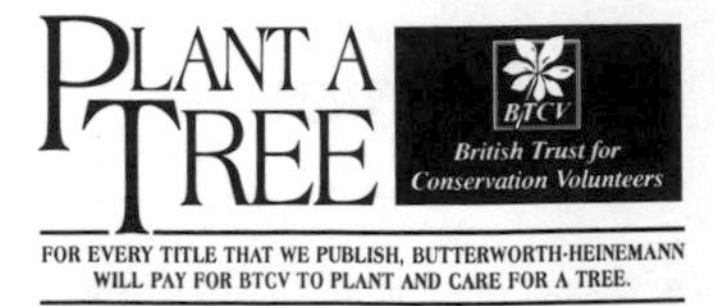

Contents

Foreword

Having willingly converted several years ago to the 'Schott and Priest' method of leading antenatal classes, I was delighted to be invited to write the Foreword to the second edition of their excellent book. Any doubts that a second edition may just be a 'tweaked' and minimally modified version of the original are quickly dispelled – this is a radically revised and thoroughly updated 'new' edition.

Certain chapters have been expanded, often to include examples of research: for instance, learning styles are explored in considerably more depth than in the original book. However, while the format and much of the detail changes, what remains in the second edition is the underlying philosophy on which the entire book is founded. Confucius is quoted as having said, 'I hear and I forget, I see and I remember, I do and I understand', and it is to this school of thought that this book's authors subscribe. For example, they state that, 'It is much easier to understand how to use new approaches when you have tried them out for yourself'. In this respect, having to commit such an interactive guide to print must have caused the authors a degree of frustration and indeed they openly acknowledge, 'the difficulty of learning a practical skill from a written text'. However, by actually doing some of the numerous exercises and activities which appear throughout the book, the reader can learn much about the reality of leading antenatal classes.

The title of the book is entirely deliberate: it is fundamentally a practical guide. The authors offer ideas for everything from adopting positive body language ('try saying "I am really delighted to be here" with a flat voice and drooping posture'), to making your own placenta and cord! The format is also very user-friendly with key points at the end of each chapter, and numerous examples of cross-referencing.

The publication of this book is particularly timely – there is currently a great deal of public interest in all aspects of maternity care, and most especially in preparation of couples for parenthood. The importance of promoting health during pregnancy and in the early years of life is becoming ever more apparent, and government funding is being channelled into several new initiatives which support such health promotion. When Judith and Judy published *Leading Antenatal Classes* in 1991,

Anne Rider in the Foreword described it as 'visionary' – and so it was. This second edition builds on their vision, using feedback from the thousands of health professionals they have met over the last ten years to improve and enrich the text.

I thoroughly recommend this book to all health professionals – even if you are not actually leading antenatal classes, you will find it useful as a quick reference guide for all aspects of maternity care. You can also use this book in the comfortable knowledge that it was written to benefit women and their families – check out the Dedication!

Lynne Pacanowski
Midwife Manager, St Mary's Hospital, Paddington, London and Lecturer in Midwifery, King's College, London

Acknowledgements

This book reflects what we know about leading antenatal classes and about ourselves as leaders. Many people have contributed to our development and understanding, and we are deeply grateful to each and every one of them.

Every page in this book reflects the PROSPECT approach, and we are indebted to Nancy James and Veronica Taylor, the partners with whom we set up PROSPECT in 1987. Working together to develop and run training workshops for health professionals was stimulating, fun and challenging, and it provided strong foundations for this book.

We would also like to thank the following people who, in one way or another, have helped us with this book. They are: Fred Adelmann, Chloe Beazley, Melissa Callaghan, Ann Keogh, Annie Hutton, Louise Long, Margaret Magnall, Vicky Manning, Lynne Pacanoswki, Sinead Saunders, Geoff Schott and Tamsin Wilton. A special thank you goes to Alix Henley, whose comments on style and clarity have, as always, been tactful and brilliant.

We are also grateful to King's College London for permission to use their library, and to the more than helpful staff at MIDIRS.

Above all, we would like to express our deep appreciation for the several thousand health professionals who have attended PROSPECT workshops throughout the UK, and shared with us their experience, skills, ideas and needs. Working with them and receiving their feedback has had a powerful influence on our thinking and approach, and has had a direct impact on this edition of our book.

Introduction

This book is written primarily for health professionals, because they teach the vast majority of parents who attend antenatal classes. Since we wrote the first edition, we have learned a great deal more about health professionals' needs and concerns. So this edition is based not only on our own experience of leading antenatal classes, but also on our work with several thousand health professionals who have attended PROSPECT workshops throughout the UK. It includes some new issues and discusses others in greater detail, giving references throughout.

The title *Leading Antenatal Classes* reflects our philosophy and practice. We believe that participants are best served by a sensitive leader who develops and maintains a creative learning environment and encourages participation. A teacher, in the strict dictionary definition of the word, is 'one who instructs'. No one denies the need to give information to new parents, but so much more than instruction can go on when a group of parents work together, talk together and get to know each other. We therefore use the word 'leader' rather than 'teacher', and, with apologies to men who lead classes, we sometimes refer to the leader as 'she'.

The second half of our title, *A practical guide*, reflects the second characteristic of this book. The book is mainly about the practical process of leading classes; how to start a group, how to get people talking, how to share information, how to teach relaxation. We acknowledge the difficulty of learning a practical skill from written text. It is much easier to understand how to use new approaches when you have seen someone else use them, and when you have tried them out for yourself. Some of our descriptions of how to do things may seem over-complicated on first reading. However, the written word is the best we can offer. You will find it easier to translate words into action if you take time to try things out, step by step, with colleagues or friends.

There are as many different ways of putting a course together as there are leaders and different groups have different needs, so we are not prescriptive about what to include. However, we do offer suggestions on how to decide on content. You will notice as you read that, like an effective antenatal class, there is overlap and some repetition. Issues don't fit into separate boxes labelled 'group work' or 'discussion' or 'teaching aids'. Topics tend to flow into one another, and can be combined in an infinite variety of new and exciting ways. So while we have divided up the material into separate topics, we often invite you to refer to other chapters as you read.

In an antenatal course, there is always more that one could include than there is room for. In the same way, we have had to make hard decisions about how much to include in this book and how much to leave out. The issues we include do not add up to a hard-and-fast recipe for running classes, but they set out what we and many others have tried and tested and found to work in practice. We hope you enjoy trying them out for yourself.

Chapter 1

The changes that pregnancy brings

Any pregnancy, but most especially a first, is a major life event. It is a time of heightened awareness and great change. Parents begin to see themselves, each other and the world differently. During the nine months it takes for a baby to grow, parents develop and grow too, so that one year later almost nothing in the parents' lives remains as it was before the baby was conceived.

Physical changes are perhaps most evident, and a woman has little choice but to take notice of them. This may be a new experience as, although most women work hard to try to ensure that their appearance conforms with current fashion and social images, many pay little real heed to their bodies. Other changes are just as intrusive and unavoidable as the growing baby forces parents to review every aspect of their lifestyles. Some are relatively trivial but may still be hard to cope with: What should the woman wear as her shape changes? Is it safe for her to continue riding her bike? What about holidays? Wine? Nightclubs? Others are more central, as they touch work, money or housing issues: Can we afford to live here? Is there room for a baby? Who will be the main carer, or do we need two incomes? What about the rising damp? Will the council give us a flat now?

Even the structure of a woman's day changes. Tiredness may force her to bed early. Broken nights and vivid dreams may find her awake at new times. Giving up work, even temporarily, is a major step. It may be a relief, but she has to adjust to the loss of a familiar routine and regular contact with friends at work. She may be anxious about stepping off the career ladder and about loss of status and income. If she plans or needs to return to full- or part-time work, she may be worried about finding affordable childcare.

It is not just practical issues. Ideas and feelings change, too. Pregnancy often seems to take the 'emotional lid' off, allowing both women and men to become more sensitive and aware. Women tend to laugh and cry more easily, whilst many men feel anxious and unsettled.

Some women cope with all the changes of pregnancy on their own, but most share the experience with a partner. The demands that pregnancy makes on the partner are often unrecognized and unacknowledged because nothing visible is happening to him. However, his world is changing too as he adapts to the physical and emotional changes in his partner, and to the financial, practical and emotional responsibilities that fatherhood brings.

Other family members will be making adjustments as well. A couple's parents may welcome or hate the idea of becoming grandparents. Some are supportive and encouraging while others may be critical, offering inappropriate advice or unwanted opinions. Some have difficulty in acknowledging that their own child is now an adult who has a demonstrably active sex life and will make his or her own decisions about the coming baby. Other family members may welcome or resent the couple's changing status and lifestyle. Whatever the attitudes, parents need to work out new ways of relating to familiar people.

Expectant parents often reassess their friendships. They may find that they have less in common with friends who do not have children. Friends with babies or small children can become role models and sources of support. Less helpfully, experienced parents may also offer conflicting or intrusive advice.

During pregnancy, parents are adapting physically and emotionally to take on what is probably the greatest responsibility of their lives. It is little wonder that, after a few months of experiencing a combination of novelty, unpredictability and discomfort, parents begin to wonder what has hit them. Where is the familiar world and their familiar part in it? Where, even, is the body they used to know? Nine months can seem endless, but it is really quite a short time in which to develop ways of coping with so much that is new.

Normal pregnancy is inherently stressful because parents are coping with so many changes within a relatively short space of time. Holmes and Rahe (1967) demonstrated the cumulative effects of stress by allocating points to various life events; the higher the score, the greater the stress. A score of 150–199 within a 12-month period equals a mild life crisis, 200–299 within a 12-month period indicates a moderate life crisis, and a score of over 300 is a major life crisis. Not everyone will agree with the precise number of points allocated to different life events, but they provide a useful baseline for reflection and demonstrate the degree of stress that commonly occurs in a normal pregnancy (see Table 1.1).

Parents adjust in all kinds of ways. Some carry on as if nothing much is happening and try to maintain life as it was before. Others seem to focus entirely on the coming baby. They may read anything they can lay their hands on, talk to experienced people, or live for their check-ups. One common strategy for coping with the changes and challenges of pregnancy is to attend antenatal classes.

Table 1.1 Having a baby (adapted from Holmes and Rahe, 1967)

Pregnancy	40
Gaining a new family member	39
Sexual difficulties	39
Change in financial status	38
Outstanding personal achievement	28
'Wife' begins or stops work	26
Change in living conditions	25
Revision of personal habits	24
Change in social activities	18
Change in sleeping habits	16
Change in eating habits	15
TOTAL	308

References

Holmes, T. H. and Rahe, R. H. (1967). The Social Adjustment Rating Scale. *Journal of Psychosomatic Research*, **11**(2), 213–18.

Chapter 2

Meeting the needs of expectant parents

This chapter reflects on what parents want from classes, and discusses the advantages and disadvantages of different approaches to parent education.

What do parents want from classes?

People come to classes for their own personal reasons. They bring with them a lifetime of experience, their own personal history, and a variety of hopes and fears. Some people see classes as a sort of rite of passage that marks their new status as expectant parents and provides them with an opportunity to focus on birth and on becoming a parent. Others come simply because it is the done thing. Some people fear that not coming would be in some way neglecting their baby or maybe even tempting fate.

Many expectant parents come to meet and talk with other people in the same situation. In everyday life, contact with pregnant women, expectant fathers or young babies is pretty unusual until one's own first baby is born. Good antenatal classes provide an introduction to peers who can exchange information, discuss anxieties and learn from each other. At their best, antenatal classes foster lasting, supportive friendships (Shearer, 1993; Cliff and Deery, 1997; Nolan, 1997, 1999).

Parents also come for information. Of course, not everybody wants exactly the same amount of detail. Some people want to know absolutely everything, while others do not want to hear 'anything gory'. Some prefer to know little or nothing – for some, this is a reason not to come to classes at all. Most people fall between these extremes and want balanced, honest and realistic information so that they know what to expect and can make informed decisions (Niven, 1992; Nolan, 1994, 1999). Many women hope for a magic formula to make their labour safe and painless, or that classes will help their partner to be supportive during labour. Some also want to increase their confidence and to learn skills that will help them feel in control of their behaviour during labour (Brewin and Bradley, 1982; Green *et al.*, 1990).

Many parents want to know about the social, emotional and psychological aspects of birth and parenting, and, contrary to the assumptions of many health professionals, most parents are keen to learn about life after birth and how to care for their babies (Coombes and Schonveld, 1992, p. 21; O'Meara, 1993; Cliff and Deery, 1997; Nolan, 1999; Singh and Newburn, 2000).

Parents may not always be fully aware of all their motives for coming to classes. Whilst many know that they have come to meet people who share their experiences and preoccupations, they may be less aware that they are also looking for behaviour patterns that they can copy, or useful information that they can tap. Another underlying reason for coming to classes may be to find family substitutes, especially if the parents' own extended family lives far away or if relationships are difficult. Even when family bonds are strong, rapid changes in midwifery and obstetric practice limit the amount of information and shared experience that older relatives can offer.

In places where continuity of clinical care is an aspiration rather than a reality, a class leader who is present throughout the antenatal course may be the only health professional who is constant, available and willing to listen. She may take on the role of an experienced woman, able to act as ally, supportive friend and information source.

Meeting parents' needs

In practice, there is often a wide discrepancy between what parents want from antenatal classes and what they get (Green *et al.*, 1990; Coombes and Schonveld, 1992, pp. 30–35; Cliff and Deery, 1997; Nolan, 1999). Why is this? Most health professionals involved in parent education are highly motivated and keen to do a good job, and there are many talented and effective class leaders. However, there are several factors that make it difficult for health professionals to lead classes effectively.

The profile of parent education

A great deal of social and political importance is attached to preparation for parenthood, but the rhetoric is not matched by resources. A survey of the views of over 1000 midwives found that they ranked parent education only seventh in the list of their duties (Kelly, 1998).

Staff shortages, budget restrictions and pressure to deliver high standards of clinical care all place great demands on maternity services. Classes tend to suffer. Class leaders often have little or no time to prepare, many teach in poor surroundings, and may face classes of up to 60 people. Some lead only one or two classes in a course and never get a chance to know or to make real contact with the parents in the class. Some health professionals end up leading classes in their own time. Even skilled and dedicated class leaders find it hard to meet parents' needs when faced with such constraints:

> *Staff are under such pressure and parent education is always the first thing to be dumped because it is seen by some as an add-on extra rather than as an essential part of maternity care.*
>
> (North West Midwives Parent and Health Education Group)

The quality of antenatal education is unlikely to improve until sufficient resources are devoted to it.

Training and support

Most health professionals receive little or no training for leading antenatal classes either as undergraduates (Kelly, 1998) or when qualified. They are often thrown in at the deep end and expected to do a good job, working on their own with little or no help or support. It is hardly surprising that some health professionals are reluctant to lead classes, or that classes often fail to meet parents' needs. It would be shocking and a cause of public outrage if so little attention was paid to preparing health professionals for any other aspect of their work. Anyone who is expected to lead classes needs training in the principles of adult education, in interactive learning techniques, and in communication and group skills. They should also have regular time to reflect, share ideas and to solve problems with their colleagues (Underdown, 1998).

Joined-up services

Parents want and expect a strong link between what they learn in classes and the support, help and care they receive in practice (Nolan, 1994; Leeseberg Stamler, 1998). This is a very reasonable expectation, but it is unlikely to be fulfilled if the professionals who care for parents during and after labour have no idea what the same parents have learnt in classes.

In addition, a course of classes, however good, cannot be a complete preparation for the stresses and challenges of labour and parenting. People cannot think clearly and may become forgetful when they are stressed, in pain or in new and unfamiliar situations. They need reminders, encouragement and active support.

The professionals who provide care during labour and afterwards may not lead classes, but they should be familiar with what is taught, and be able to enhance and support women's ability to apply what they have learned and to teach women who have not been to classes. Meeting parents' needs means providing a seamless service. If classes are run in isolation from the rest of maternity services, effectiveness is reduced and parents are likely to feel let down.

Philosophy and approach

There is no universally agreed definition of the aims of antenatal classes. Consequently there is a wide variety of styles, based on different assumptions about what classes are for. Some classes encourage parents to be passive, accepting and dependent on 'experts'. Others encourage them to see themselves as competent and able to make informed choices for themselves and for their baby – something that will be expected of them from the time they take their child home until he or she is grown up!

Below we discuss the potentials of different approaches to antenatal education.

Education or clinical care?

Some class leaders treat the antenatal course as an extension of clinical care. This may be due to lack of preparation and training for class leadership, and it may be the only approach they have ever seen. However, it has several drawbacks; proven principles of effective adult education are often ignored, and there is a danger that the class leader will control the content, present all the information, give instructions and be the sole focus of attention. Parents' feelings may be ignored, opportunities for discussion omitted, and their concerns not be addressed (see Chapter 3).

In some places, topics such as diet and dental care are included in classes. If these topics are covered in antenatal care, precious time is lost if they are repeated in classes. Conversely, if essential topics are not part of antenatal care, the most vulnerable (who are also likely to have poorer outcomes) will miss out because they are the least likely to come to classes.

Course planners and class leaders need to make a clear distinction between:

- clinical care, including information that is essential for the safety and well being of the mother and baby and
- antenatal classes, which are optional and which should be an educational opportunity.

Predetermined learning outcomes

Devising learning outcomes is an accepted part of planning and delivering many education programmes. However, some people argue that this approach is too directive and therefore not universally appropriate (Rogers, 2000). Predetermined outcomes are bound to reflect the objectives of the leader or the programme planners, and may ignore parents' needs and aspirations. Identifying learning outcomes assumes that it is possible to check what people have learned and how they will apply it. However, outcomes may well not be evident for weeks, months or even years. Most experienced class leaders have met someone years later who says that classes made such a difference to them, and they have never forgotten what they learned.

Advice or information?

Expectant parents are sometimes regarded as a captive audience for health education advice and messages, and classes seen as a golden opportunity for influencing their beliefs and actions (Braun and Schonveld, 1993). It is easy to feel justified in giving strong messages about what a woman should and should not do when her actions will affect not just herself, but also the baby that she is carrying and will be caring for the next decade or two. Helping women to stop smoking and avoid teratogens and unnecessary stress brings real benefits to mother and baby. Posture, diet and dental care come under the 'good for the mother' label, whilst vaccination, breastfeeding and effective car restraints are 'good for the baby'.

Although it is true that most expectant parents think about how they care for themselves and how they plan to care for their baby, the impetus for actual changes in behaviour has to come from within. It is clear from the results of numerous health education programmes that human beings do not blindly follow advice (Hollins, 2000). There is a tenuous link between knowing that something is harmful or beneficial, and acting on that knowledge. Do you and your colleagues consistently put into practice everything you know is good for your own health?

People make their own decisions about whether or not to take advice. Some resist advice on principle. Some avoid antenatal classes because they do not want to be told what they should do. Others may have every intention of acting on the advice they are given, but for a range of personal reasons and circumstances find it too difficult.

Advice that does not acknowledge individuals' situations and difficulties is a burden, not an asset. It alienates. So too does an implicit message that equates failure to follow advice with irresponsibility. The additional stress and guilt may even cause people to increase the behaviour that the message was designed to change.

Advice is sometimes appropriate in clinical settings because it can be tailored to the person's individual needs and combined with appropriate support. However, there are several reasons to be very cautious about giving advice in antenatal classes:

- the assumption that antenatal classes are an effective way of changing attitudes and behaviour is not borne out by research. Studies indicate that most women have made up their minds about issues such as pain relief in labour and infant feeding long before they come to classes (OPCS, 1992; Nolan, 2000)
- advice given to a group of people is likely to come across as directive and patronising, and to alienate rather than motivate them

- advice is unlikely to be followed unless it is tailored to the individual's situation and combined with support.

Effective class leaders distinguish between:

- *information* about the pros and cons of a course of action so that people can make informed choices, and
- *advice*, that is, telling people what they should do.

Maintaining the status quo

Sometimes the goal of classes is to prepare parents for what they will actually meet in labour or on the postnatal ward. How would you teach your class if you knew, despite the evidence that routine continuous electronic fetal monitoring gives no advantage to many women and babies and is associated with a higher intervention rate, that all the women attending your class would be attached to an electronic fetal monitor? Is there any point in encouraging people to practise a variety of positions in classes so that they can remain mobile throughout labour, if you know that this is not encouraged on the labour ward? How will you broach the issue of making choices if you know that, in practice, labour ward protocols and policies tend to prevail?

Whether by choice or under pressure, some class leaders teach to maintain the *status quo*. Not doing so can lead to serious difficulties with colleagues, managers and obstetricians. Raising parents' awareness of what might be possible can also mean that they come back disappointed and upset after the birth because their experience fell short of their expectations.

However, teaching for compliance also denies parents the information they have a right to, and deprives them of opportunities to make choices for themselves and their babies. It turns them into passive recipients of care. It encourages dependence and reliance on experts at the expense of developing parents' confidence in the innate ability of a woman's body to nurture and give birth to her baby, and in themselves as responsible parents. Handling these conflicting pressures is not easy. However, if the principles and approaches used in classes are evidence-based, they should also be applied in clinical care although it may take time, tact and persistence to effect change (see Chapter 23).

Challenging the status quo

Some class leaders believe that encouraging parents to challenge the system is a good way to improve maternity services. There is no doubt that consumer pressure has changed the face of maternity care. The 1982 march on the Royal Free Hospital in London certainly shocked the obstetric and midwifery establishment of the day into change (Ferriman, 1982). However, this only happens when a sufficient number of people band together, and the effects are sometimes disappointingly short-lived.

Supporting parents in the choices they make is one thing; expecting them to monitor or change the system during their own pregnancy and labour is asking a great deal of people at a time when they are vulnerable and dependent.

Persuasion and charismatic teaching

Some class leaders influence parents by offering their own personal beliefs and convictions, for example about high-tech obstetrics, 'natural' childbirth, excluding men, involving siblings at the birth, water birth, or any other approach about which they feel strongly. Because expectant parents are anxious, eager for knowledge and unsure of themselves, they may be persuaded to adapt their behaviour to match the convictions of a charismatic teacher.

Persuasive and charismatic teachers genuinely believe their way is best. They want parents to benefit from their experience, which often comes from years of practice or work with hundreds of couples. At one level this makes good sense – after all, there is a reason why a professional or trained layperson runs classes rather than the milkman!

However, charisma and persuasion do not offer parents a balanced picture. Most firmly held beliefs can be challenged with an opposite viewpoint that someone else holds just as tenaciously – for example, 'home birth is the best' or 'it's safer in hospital'; 'labour without an epidural? What's the point of feeling pain?' or 'drugs for pain mean a second-rate labour and a second-rate start for your baby'. None of these statements is an absolute truth, and only individual parents can judge which option is best for them. A class leader who offers strong convictions may believe that she is giving others the benefits she herself has found. In practice this approach benefits her, rather than the parents.

Patchwork classes

A patchwork course is one where different parts of the course are led by health professionals from different disciplines. In some places strict boundaries define who teaches what, and occasionally demarcation disputes arise. For parents this can result in a disjointed and fragmented course in which certain topics are duplicated and others omitted. When staff from different disciplines teach the same group, it is essential that they establish a common philosophy and approach, and that they plan the course together. They also need to review and communicate on a regular basis (see Chapter 18).

Parent-centred classes

Parent-centred classes foster social support, confidence and choice. The principles of adult learning are observed, parents participate in setting the agenda, and the leader creates a learning environment that enables people to talk about what really matters to them.

We wrote this book because we believe that parent-centred classes are the most effective and the most fun for both parents and class leaders. As you read, there may be times when you feel that, however much you want to, it is quite impossible for you to work in some of the ways we suggest. We realize that resources and the scope for change are often limited. You may be leading classes in difficult circumstances, and be under a variety of constraints. If so, you may not be able to make all the changes you want overnight. It may take time and patience to achieve your goals (see Chapter 21). However, we make no apology for being idealistic and setting out the very best we know. Without a vision, nothing great is likely to be achieved.

Key points

- Research into antenatal education indicates that parents' needs and expectations are not being met.
- Lack of resources and staff training reduce the potential of antenatal education.
- There is a lack of clarity about the purpose of antenatal education.
- A variety of approaches are used, some of which fail to meet parents' needs.
- A parent-centred approach which takes the principles of adult learning into account is likely to be the most effective.

References

Brewin, C. and Bradley, C. (1982). Perceived control and the experience of childbirth. *British Journal of Clinical Psychology*, **21**, 263–9.

Braun, D. and Schonveld, A. (1993). *Approaching Parenthood: A Resource for Parent Education*, p. 11. Health Education Authority.

Cliff, D. and Deery, R. (1997). Too much like school; social class, age, marital status and attendance/non-attendance at antenatal classes. *Midwifery*, **13**, 139–45.

Coombes, G. and Schonveld, A. (1992). *Life Will Never be the Same Again*. Health Education Authority.

Ferriman, A. (1982). 5000 join natural childbirth rally. *The Times*, 5th April, p. 2.

Green, J. M., Kitzinger, J. V. and Coupland, V. A. (1990). Stereotypes of childbearing women: a look at some evidence. *Midwifery*, **6**, 125–32.

Hollins, C. (2000). Knowledge about attitudes can help change behaviour. *British Journal of Midwifery*, **8**(11), 690–94.

Kelly, S. (1998). Parenting education survey. *RCM Midwives Journal*, **1**(1), 23–5.

Leeseberg Stamler, L. (1998). The participants' view of childbirth education: is there congruency with an ennoblement framework for patient education? *Journal of Advanced Nursing*, **28**(5), 939–47.
Niven, C. A. (1992). *Psychological Care for Families Before, During and After Birth*, pp. 61–3. Butterworth-Heinemann.
Nolan, M. (1994). Effectiveness of parent education. *British Journal of Midwifery*, **2**(11), 534–8.
Nolan, M. (1997). Antenatal education – where next? *Journal of Advanced Nursing*, **25**, 1198–1204.
Nolan, M. (1999). Antenatal education: past and future agendas. *The Practising Midwife*, **2**(3), 24–6.
Nolan, M. (2000). The influence of antenatal classes on pain relief in labour: a review of the literature. *The Practising Midwife*, **3**(5), 23–31.
O'Meara, C. (1993). An evaluation of consumer perspectives of childbirth and parenting education. *Midwifery*, **9**, 10–219.
OPCS (1992) *Infant Feeding*. Office of Populations Censuses and Surveys, Social Services Division, HMSO.
Rogers, A. (2000). *Teaching Adults*, p. 117. Open University Press.
Shearer, H. (1993). Commentary: effects of prenatal classes cannot be measured by obstetric management. *Birth*, **20**, 130–1.
Singh, D. and Newburn, M. (2000). *Becoming a Father: Men's Access to Information and Support about Pregnancy, Birth and Life with a New Baby*. The National Childbirth Trust.
Underdown, A. (1998). Investigating techniques used in parenting classes. *Health Visitor*, **71**(2), 65–8.

Chapter 3

How people learn

This chapter summarizes the factors that contribute to effective adult learning. The following chapters describe, in detail, ways of putting these factors into practice.

Human beings are born with an enormous enthusiasm and capacity to learn. You have only to watch babies and very young children to see that human beings are inherently alert and deeply interested in and inquisitive about themselves, other people and the world around them. This capacity and enthusiasm for learning can be enhanced by positive learning experiences, or dampened by negative ones.

Starting with yourself

Before reading on, take a few minutes to reflect on your own experiences of learning. Think about the best teacher or teachers you ever had. Don't restrict yourself to teachers you had at school or during your professional training. You come into contact with a whole variety of people in very different circumstances – some of these may have been the key people from whom you learnt most. Now list all the qualities, the things they did and said, that made them such a good teacher for you. Then think about the worst teacher you ever had, and list the things they said and did that made learning difficult.

Now focus on your learning experiences as an adult:

- Write down one or two new skills you have acquired in the last couple of years.
- What was your motivation for learning these?
- What kept you going?
- What approaches and methods helped you to learn?
- Do you absorb information and acquire skills by listening, watching, reading, discussing or experimenting?

Invite some of your friends and colleagues to do this exercise too. Your combined lists will help you identify the different ways that individuals learn, and some of the behaviours and attitudes that assist learning and those that do not.

Creating a climate for learning

A great deal is now known about the factors that contribute to a creative learning environment for adults. You can compare them with the factors that have enabled you to learn.

The characteristics of adult learners

> *Knowledge is not the preserve of the few, the educated to be doled out in small parcels to ... participants. It is something we can all share in creating and discovering, which we all view from our own particular perspective.*
> (Rogers, 2000, p. 237)

Adults are not empty vessels waiting to be filled. They share certain characteristics. Adults:

- are experienced
- are in a continuous process of learning and growing
- already know a great deal
- have many demands on their time and attention
- choose to come to classes for their own personal reasons
- bring with them a set of expectations, values, assumptions and beliefs
- each has his or her own preferred ways of learning (Rogers, 2000, pp. 60–70).

To be effective, adult education needs to acknowledge and work with these characteristics. It should also promote personal growth and a sense of perspective, autonomy and responsibility (Rogers, 2000, p. 36).

The hierarchy of needs

According to Maslow (1970), there is a hierarchy of needs that are shared by all human beings. Each level of need must be met, starting with the most fundamental, before a person is able to move on to the next level of need. The primary need is for physiological wellbeing; the second is the need for safety and security; the third is the need to belong and feel accepted; and the fourth need is for esteem – that is, to be recognized, approved of and to feel competent. This hierarchy of needs has important implications for antenatal classes.

The environment
In order to learn, people need to feel at ease. They need comfort and privacy in order to relax and focus on the job in hand. This has implications for the venue and the facilities that are available.

Safety and respect
People will be more able to listen, think and try new things if there is an atmosphere of mutual respect and acceptance for every single person in the class, whatever their knowledge, views, background or lifestyle. People also learn best from someone they respect and trust. These feelings are not conferred automatically; they have to be earned. This makes continuity of class leader or leaders essential.

The human attention span and the importance of variety

Several studies have shown that length of time that students can listen to and retain information is between 15 and 25 minutes (Barrington, 1965; Wood and Hedley, 1968; MacManaway, 1970). Mills (1996) found that limited attention applied to educational television programmes as well as to lectures. The average person's attention span is therefore around 20 minutes. After this, people's ability to listen to and absorb new information declines rapidly. Pregnancy amnesia probably reduces this span considerably, and is likely to affect women's ability to concentrate and to remember what they have heard (Sharp *et al.*, 1993; Stark, 2000).

This means that there is no point in talking at length. However, you can keep people alert and interested if, in each class, you continuously alternate:

- *information* – that is, things people want or need to know, with
- *physical skills* – for example, relaxation, positions for labour, pelvic floor exercises, positioning a baby at the breast and with
- *attitudes and feelings* – this includes small group discussion, reflection and time for people to discover and try things out for themselves.

Learning styles

Another reason for using variety is that people learn in different ways. (Rogers, 2000, pp. 70–71). There are no universally accepted definitions of the variety of learning styles (Curry, 1990), which are influenced by a range of factors including culture and personality (Furnham, 1992; Jones, 1998). This means that in every class people will have different learning styles. People may prefer to listen, to see things, to take notes or to read. Most people find it helpful to discuss, question or experiment. If you use a variety of techniques and keep changing your approach throughout each class, you offer everyone an opportunity to learn in their own particular way.

A shared agenda

People are more motivated if they play a part in deciding what they will learn (Rogers, 2000, p. 86). This is very different from transferring a predetermined body of knowledge or skills into passive recipients. Parents will have more investment in the course if they have helped to set the agenda and class leaders are more likely to meet the parents needs (see Chapters 5 and 16).

Building on existing knowledge

People find it easier to grasp a new idea if it relates in some way to something they already understand. By encouraging them to identify what they already know, you boost their self-esteem and build a sound foundation for new skills and knowledge. You benefit too, because understanding what they already know helps you to give information in a way that is appropriate to the people with whom you are working (see Chapter 9).

Establishing relevance

People are motivated to learn if they can see some personal relevance or advantage in making the effort (Strong, 1996; Jarvis and Gibson, 1997; Dearling, 1999). People who do not see any benefit in learning about a topic may look attentive, but in reality they are likely to spend the time thinking 'what is the point of this?' or 'this doesn't apply to me'. If you identify and include the things that people want from the course and take time to establish why additional topics, information and skills would also be useful, you stimulate people's willingness to learn. One way of establishing relevance and benefit is to identify skills and information that could be useful in everyday life as well as in childbearing (see Chapters 6, 11 and 12).

Carrots not sticks

Salespeople and advertisers are in the business of motivating people and changing behaviour. They know that in order to succeed, they must show how their product will benefit the client. Dearling (1999) compares the art of selling with the way information about health is given. Selling focuses on the 'what's in it for me?' factor. Taking breastfeeding as his topic, Dearling observes that health professionals tend to focus on the benefits for the baby. This approach relies on parental altruism and ignores the concerns and feelings of the mother and her partner. It can also engender guilt. In short, it is a stick, not a carrot.

Many of the issues covered in classes sound like sticks and are therefore off-putting. However, with a little thought they can be converted into carrots, which stimulate interest and motivation. Which of the following sound more inviting:

- 'posture and lifting in pregnancy' or 'avoiding and easing backache'?
- 'the role of the midwife and health visitor' or 'who you can contact for help and advice'?
- 'why breastfeeding is best for your baby' or 'what advantages breast-feeding has for mothers and fathers'?
- 'the postnatal period' or 'life after birth'?

Bridging the expectation–experience gap

Objective facts do not prepare people for the subjective experience. People who do not have realistic expectations of an event can feel devastated by what actually happens (Niven, 1992). If you prepare people for the physical and emotional realities of labour and early parenthood, when the time comes they will know that what they are experiencing is normal. If you offer coping strategies, they are more able to help themselves.

Encouragement and affirmation

Success breeds success. Everyone becomes more confident, relaxed and able to learn if each person's contributions and efforts, no matter how small, are appreciated. When people are rewarded with encouragement, they will often risk a bigger step in future. Criticism that usually focuses on what is wrong has the opposite effect on motivation and morale. If you avoid situations in which there is a right or wrong answer and 'adjust' inaccurate information with sensitivity and respect, you reduce the chances of people feeling criticized (see Chapter 9).

Learning can be fun

For many of us learning has been a fraught and serious business. However, fun and learning are not mutually exclusive. Some of the most effective learning and most creative work takes place when people are enjoying each other's company and having fun together.

Key points

Where human beings are concerned, nothing is ever guaranteed or fool-proof. However, research and experience demonstrate that people are likely to get the most out of classes if you:

- get the welcome right
- create safety by demonstrating respect and helping people to feel part of the group

- establish the class members' agenda and meet it
- offer carrots not sticks
- change the format frequently; intersperse 'information' with 'physical skills' and 'attitudes and feelings'
- use approaches that allow people to see, to do and to reflect
- bridge the information–experience gap.

References

Barrington, H. (1965). A survey of instructional television researches. *Educational Research*, **18**(1), 8–25. Cited in Bligh, D. (1998). *What's the Use of Lectures?*, 3rd edn, p. 53. Intellect.

Curry, L. (1990). A critique of the research on learning styles. *Educational Leadership*, **48**(2), 50–56.

Dearling, J. (1999). The carrot and its role in the promotion of breastfeeding. *The Practising Midwife*, **2**(1), 19–20.

Furnham, A.(1992). Personality and learning style: a study of three instruments. *Personality and Individual Differences*, **4**, 429–38.

Jarvis, P. and Gibson, S. (1997). *The Teacher Practitioner and Mentor in Nursing, Midwifery Health Visiting and Social Services*, 2nd edn, p. 77. Stanley Thorsons.

Jones, S. (1998). Learning styles and learning strategies. *Forum for Modern Language Studies*, **34**(2), 114–29.

MacManaway, L. A. (1970). Teaching methods in higher education – innovation and research. *Universities Quarterly*, **24**(3), 53, 137, 163, 321–9. Cited in Bligh, D. (1998). *What's the Use of Lectures?*, 3rd edn, p. 53. Intellect.

Maslow, A. (1970). *Motivation and Personality*, 3rd edn, pp. 15–22. Harper Row Publishers.

Mills, D. G. (1996). The use of closed circuit television in teaching geography. *Geography*, **51**(3), 203, 319–25. Cited in Bligh, D. (1998). *What's the Use of Lectures?*, 3rd edn, p. 53. Intellect.

Niven, C. A. (1992). *Psychological Care for Families Before, During and After Birth*, pp. 59–61. Butterworth-Heinemann.

Rogers, A. (2000). *Teaching Adults*. Open University Press.

Sharp, K., Brindle, P. M., Brown, M. W. and Turner, G. (1993). Memory loss during pregnancy. *British Journal of Obstetrics and Gynaecology*, **100**(3), 209–15.

Stark, M. A. (2000). Is it difficult to concentrate during the third trimester and postpartum? *Journal of Obstetric, Gynecologic and Neonatal Nursing*, **29**(4), 378–89.

Strong, T. (1996). Tennis balls and prostitutes. What can health care learn from advertising? *King's Fund News*, **19**(3), 4.

Wood, C. C. and Hedley, R. L. (1968). Student reaction to VTR in simulated classroom conditions. *Canadian Educational Research Digest*, **8**(1), 46–59. Cited in Bligh, D. (1998). *What's the Use of Lectures?*, 3rd edn, p. 53. Intellect.

Chapter 4

Being a class leader

This chapter is about you, the class leader. It discusses the leader's role, the importance of reflection, ways of managing first impressions, and ways to build and maintain confidence.

What is a leader?

You may or may not think of yourself as a leader, but if you lead classes that is what you are. Parents rely on you for information. You are a resource, someone who has an understanding of their situation and someone they may choose as a role model.

People come with ready-made attitudes to leaders. These stem from their assumptions about leaders and from previous experiences of being led. Some people are very deferential and anxious to please the leader. Others expect the leader to be perfect and to have the answer to everything. Some may be competitive, suspicious or antagonistic.

You too may make assumptions about what leading actually involves. There is a tendency to believe that the leader is totally responsible for everything and everybody and has to get everything right. Health professionals sometimes confuse class leadership with their clinical responsibilities. Leaders may feel they ought to be separate and different. Many leaders work in relative isolation – indeed this may feel safer and more comfortable, because when other leaders are around feelings of inadequacy or competitiveness may creep in.

Leadership does indeed carry responsibilities – for example, your primary role is to ensure that the people in your group achieve their goals (Adair, 1988). However, some of the assumptions about leading are unrealistic and unhelpful. This is not surprising, since many leaders, both current and historical, are associated with power and control, or appear to be superhuman and set apart from ordinary people.

Different leadership styles are commonly defined as autocratic, democratic or *laissez faire* (Guirdham, 1990, p. 363). Leaders may have a preferred style, but effective leaders use different styles to deal with different needs. For example, skilful class leaders are democratic in that they create a warm, safe environment. They are respectful and responsive, and aim to empower other people. They ensure that the aims of the group are achieved. At times they are autocratic in that they take the initiative and, where necessary, take charge. On occasions they may be *laissez faire* in that they allow time for the unexpected, letting discussion evolve or dealing with unplanned topics. They may then need to revert to an autocratic style to get back on track. What is your preferred leadership style? Are you able to use different styles for different situations?

Effective leaders also know their limitations and are able to admit to them. They do not set themselves apart. They take time to reflect on what they do and how they do it, and to evaluate and develop their skills. They know how to *look* confident and how to create a good impression. They also ensure that their own needs for input and support are met (see Chapters 20 and 21).

The importance of reflection

Effective leaders are reflective, and throughout this book you will find invitations to think about your own attitudes. There is nothing wrong with having your own beliefs and preferences – in fact, it is inevitable. However, it is important to be aware of them, because they can strongly affect the way you lead classes. They may influence what you include and what you leave out, and affect your ability to give a balanced and objective view.

Think about all the topics and issues that are relevant to antenatal classes. Take, for example, beliefs about childbirth. On one extreme there are people who believe that it is a normal, natural process that is inhibited by modern obstetric practice. On the other, there are people who maintain that birth is potentially dangerous and should only be considered safe in retrospect. Where do you stand? Can you be objective and balance extreme views?

If you find it difficult to be objective and balanced about any topic or issue, or have especially strong feelings about it, think about why. What happened that influenced your views? Being aware of the origins of your views may or may not change them, but it can help you to set them on one side so that you can give parents a balanced view.

Making a good impression

First impressions are formed within seconds or minutes of meeting, and are important because they tend to last. People have a tendency to ignore or distort information they receive later if it does not fit with their first impression (Guirdham, 1990, p. 113; Hicks, 1993). So time and effort spent on creating a good impression when people first come to your class is an investment.

Goffman (1990) suggests that all social interactions are performances. Good class leaders play a variety of parts. They are stage managers in that they organize the setting for the class; they are hosts, giving a warm welcome; like conductors, they orchestrate what happens; and like actors, they use words and body language to communicate. You can maximize your ability to create positive first impressions in several ways.

The way you speak sends powerful messages. Listeners gain some information from what the speaker says, but the strongest impression is conveyed by the speaker's body language – the non-verbal cues such as gesture, posture, tone of voice, or facial expression. Not only is the verbal message the smallest component, it is also the first to be discounted when the body language contradicts what is being said (Guirdham, 1990, pp. 117–22). Try saying 'I am really delighted to be here' with a flat voice and drooping posture. Anyone listening to you will be confused by the inconsistent message you are sending, and will probably believe the non-verbal clues that say you are not delighted rather than the words that say you are. Posture and facial expressions are as important as intonation. People who smile, nod their heads, look at people and lean towards them when interacting are judged to be warmer and more likeable. They are also more likely to hold people's attention (Argyle, 1988).

You may not give the impression you think you give, so it is worthwhile finding out how you come across. Most people do not have opportunities to see or hear themselves as others do, and many are embarrassed about the way they assume they look and sound. Therefore, having objective information about how you come across is useful, even if the prospect of finding out about it feels daunting! You can find out about your facial expression right now. Adopt the expression you would use to greet people arriving at the first class. Now hold it, and go and look in the mirror. Do you actually look friendly and welcoming? If not, try changing your expression, *notice how it feels*, and then practise until conveying the impression you want is easy.

You can find out about the clarity and tone of your voice and about your posture by asking a sympathetic friend or colleague for feedback, by taping your voice so that you can listen to yourself, or by asking someone to video you in action. Do you look friendly, alert and interested? Do you sound clear and caring? Do you send out cues that make it easy for others to ask you questions? Do you have any distracting mannerisms? Asking for and giving this kind of feedback is not easy. The least painful approach is to ask the other person to tell you first what you do well, and then what could be improved and how. This will give you some positive feedback and some strategies for improving (see Chapter 20).

People also judge others by their clothes and grooming, so think about the impression you want to give, and dress to suit the occasion. Uniform can convey authority and competence, but can also create barriers. Casual clothes convey a more relaxed approach, but need to be neat and practical for moving and demonstrating. Anything tight and glamorous may be off-putting especially to pregnant women, who are likely to be concerned about their own body image.

Building and maintaining your confidence

Confident leaders perform better, and are more likely to inspire confidence in others. In other words, confidence is good for everyone. Being confident does not mean being arrogant or dominating; it means believing in yourself, doing as well as you can, setting realistic goals and having the ability to *act* confidently even if you don't feel it (Taylor, 2000). If the idea of leading a class is daunting, or if your confidence has recently taken a knock, you could try the following strategies.

Act confidently

When you know how your body feels and looks when you are confident, you can recreate the physical appearance of confidence even when you don't feel it. Changing your behaviour can also actually change how you feel (Guirdham, 1990, pp. 123–6), so the more you act being confident, the more likely you are to start feeling confident. Think of a time when you felt really confident, relaxed and good about yourself. Remember how you felt physically, and notice how your posture, stance and facial expression changes. Stand up and pay attention to the feeling of your feet on the ground. Notice how you hold your head and the way your face feels. Try saying 'brush', and notice how your cheek muscles lift slightly and soften your expression. Now smile! Doing this in front of a mirror gives you visual as well as sensory feedback. You could also try the standing relaxation described in Chapter 11.

Harness the self-fulfilling prophecy

Professional sportspeople are taught to visualize effectiveness and success, and the technique can work equally well for class leaders. Try replacing all the negative thoughts you have about yourself, your performance and the people in your class with positive ones. Instead of worrying or anticipating the worst, imagine yourself doing well. See yourself looking and sounding confident with a group of people who are enjoying and benefiting from your leadership. You may have to be vigilant, as old habits are hard to shift. Keep checking your thoughts, and turn anything negative into a positive.

Set realistic goals

This is especially important if you have little or no experience of leading classes. It takes time to develop new skills and new ways of working, so start off simply, focus on what you do well, and build on your successes (see Chapters 20 and 21). You do not have to be perfect, and neither do you have to have all the answers. If you cannot answer a question, say so and promise to find out and pass on the answer in the next session.

Decide where your boundaries are

People feel more comfortable about a leader if they know a little bit about her as a person. Some parents are very keen to know what the class leader would choose, and what sort of births she has had. Some health professionals are happy to respond to personal questions. However, it is important to strike a balance. A leader who says too little may seem aloof whereas one who says too much can sound self-centred; anyway, the leader's personal views and life history are not necessarily helpful to people whose experiences are likely to be different. Some leaders find such questions intrusive. They can be especially difficult for health professionals who do not have children or who have experienced childbearing losses. You may find it helpful to think about how you would feel if you were asked personal questions, and to plan how you would respond (Bewley, 2000).

Obtain training and support

Class leaders in the NHS tend to work in isolation, are seldom offered training, and rarely get together to share ideas and to support each other. However, if you are to remain effective you need time and attention. It's like looking after your bank account – if you don't make deposits, there will be trouble. You need to share ideas, update your information, review your attitudes and feelings, and assess and improve your skills (see Chapters 20 and 21). You also need to build and maintain your enthusiasm:

> *There is only one thing more contagious than enthusiasm and that's the lack of it.*
>
> (Bligh, 1998)

Key points

- It is important to examine your assumptions about leaders, and to be clear about what leadership actually involves.

- Reflection is essential, because your attitudes and beliefs can influence your ability to be balanced and objective.
- Being aware of how you come across can help you to make a good impression.
- There are several ways to build and maintain your confidence.

References

Adair, J. (1988). *Effective Leadership*, p. 77. Pan Books.

Argyle, M. (1988). *Bodily Communication*, p. 88. Routledge.

Bewley, C. (2000). Feelings and experiences of midwives who do not have children about caring for childbearing women. *Midwifery*, **16**, 135–44.

Bligh, D. (1998). *What's the Use of Lectures?*, 3rd edn, p. 63. Intellect.

Goffman, E. (1990). *The Presentation of Self in Everyday Life*, p. 28. Penguin Books.

Guirdham, M. (1990). *Interpersonal Skills at Work*. Prentice Hall.

Hicks, C. (1993). Effects of psychological prejudices on communication and social interaction. *British Journal of Midwifery*, **1**(1), 10–16.

Taylor, R. (2000). *Confidence in Just Seven Days*, p. 8. Vermilion, Ebury Press.

Chapter 5

The first class

This chapter discusses the factors that help to create a supportive learning environment, and offers practical suggestions for forming interactive learning groups and for finding out what the parents in your group want to cover.

Coming to an antenatal class can be an exciting milestone, marking the progress of pregnancy. However, like any new and unfamiliar experience, it is also likely to generate a certain amount of anxiety. Parents may be wondering 'Will I find my way?', 'Who else will be there?', 'Will I fit in?', 'What will the teacher be like?', 'What will be expected of me?'. They may also be reminded of previous learning experiences. These will be as varied as the people who come. Those whose success depended on amassing and remembering facts often see birth and parenthood like another test to pass or fail. They may want clear-cut information and a defined set of actions to follow which will produce the desired effect. Others, who found schooling competitive and learning difficult, may have an aversion to being taught or put into any situation where there is a 'right' or a 'wrong' answer. They may be fearful that their worst memories of being put on the spot or feeling humiliated will be repeated. Others are deferential and anxious to please, whilst a few will be suspicious or even antagonistic.

Anxiety interferes with people's ability to learn, so your task is to ensure that everything you do is designed to reduce tension and to help people to feel safe and comfortable. You can do this by offering a warm welcome, treating everyone with respect, never asking questions that have a right or wrong answer, and avoiding putting people on the spot. The atmosphere at the first class is especially important, because it sets the tone for the whole course. The first class is a bit like a shop window. If it is attractive, people will want to enter in more fully.

First impressions

First impressions have lasting effects on people's attitudes and responses. The impression you give starts before the parents arrive. Most of our suggestions for offering a warm welcome and creating a positive impression seem obvious – they are things none of us would dream of forgetting when we invite guests into our own homes. However, in a work environment it is all too easy to forget to do the little things that will help reduce people's anxiety when they enter a strange and new situation.

Invitations

If you advertise your classes, make sure that your handout or flyer is inviting:

- Is it addressed directly to the reader ('you are welcome' rather than 'women are welcome'?
- Do you explain what people will gain from coming?
- If men and women are invited, does every single word apply to both sexes?
- Have you been clear and accurate about the commitment – time, place and length?
- What does the style imply about the atmosphere and approach of the classes?
- Ask yourself, 'Suppose this was an invitation to a party, would I go? Does it sound interesting enough to stir me into making the effort?'
- Does the handout use large print and include plenty of white space?
- Is it clear and concise? What could be cut?
- Does it contain everyday language, or has medical language crept in?
- Are the sentences short?
- Does it describe a fixed, prescriptive programme, or does it imply a flexible and informal approach?

The venue

The environment in which you lead classes is important. People are affected, however unconsciously, by their surroundings. The setting affects the degree to which people feel that they are valued, and influences their feelings about the quality of what is on offer.

The ideal teaching room is easily accessible, clean, uncluttered, well lit and ventilated, square, private and carpeted. It has facilities for making tea and coffee, and adequate, clean lavatories for women and men nearby. The ideal chairs have padded seats and backs, no arms, can be moved easily, and are the right width to allow people to sit astride them comfortably.

Sadly, many class leaders cope with something far short of this. You may need to work to minimize the disadvantages and maximize the potential of your venue. Here are some ideas for preparing your venue before the class arrives:

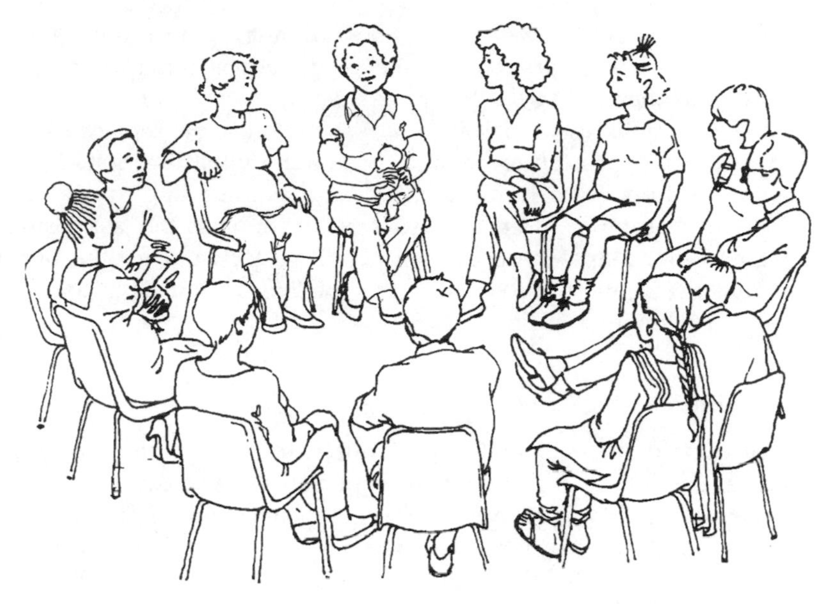

Figure 5.1

- Arrange the chairs in a circle so that everyone will be able see everyone else. If you can, have similar chairs for everyone, make the circle as round as possible, remove any tables or equipment from the middle, and include your own chair in the circle (Figure 5.1). When people return to a circle from smaller groups, they tend leave gaps or form a horseshoe shape around you as the teacher. If this happens, encourage them to 'smooth' the circle. If the circle is small in relation to the size of the room, place it near one corner. If the room is too small for one large circle, try two circles, one inside another, and move people frequently since most people feel uncomfortable sitting in the inner circle.
- If you use a flip chart, place the stand in the circle and make sure that it is not in front of a window. Light from behind makes it difficult to see what is on the chart.
- Remove clutter and outdated posters. Put unwanted, broken and unsuitable equipment out of sight.
- Have facilities for people to make their own tea and coffee in the room. If possible provide biscuits, especially at evening classes when people tend to arrive preoccupied by hunger. If you need to ask for donations to cover costs, put out a sign and a collecting box. If you use disposable cups, you will use fewer if you put out a felt-tip pen and a sign asking people to write their name on their cup.

Maps and directions

Finding one's way to somewhere new and wondering where to park generate an inordinate amount of anxiety. People who have difficulty finding the venue are likely to arrive stressed, angry and resentful, so it pays to make sure that parents receive clear directions, a map and details of parking facilities. *When designing your directions and map, ask someone who does not know the way to follow them*. When you know a place like the back of your hand, it is all too easy to miss out a vital direction.

Put up direction signs from the entrance of the building to the room, making sure that you can see the next sign as you pass the last. Using a distinctive colour helps – you can tell people to look out for the purple signs. Prop the venue door open so that people do not have to worry about opening the wrong door.

The welcome

We have found that the most effective strategy for welcoming people is to be ready at the door and to smile at each person as he or she arrives. This means arriving early to prepare the room and overcoming our own embarrassment and anxiety. However, we have discovered that the more energy we put into helping participants to feel at home, the more relaxed and confident we feel.

Show people where to hang their coats, point out the lavatories, and invite people to help themselves to a drink and biscuit and to make themselves at home.

You may need to find ways of preventing people sitting in awkward silence, especially at the start of the first class. For example, you could:

- introduce people to each other, just as you would do if you were giving a party
- offer the first arrivals sticky labels and a felt-tip pen, and suggest they write their own name badges in large letters and then pass on these instructions to the next person who comes in; organizing this often gets people talking to each other
- scatter books, leaflets, pictures, photographs or baby equipment in the centre of the circle and invite people to have a look at what is on offer.

Getting started

People are never all there by the appointed starting time, and with an open group you never know how many are coming. However, if you wait too long for stragglers you will find that the number of latecomers goes up week by week. Delaying also disregards the effort made by you and the rest of the group to come on time. The best solution is to start on time and design the first part of your session in such a way as to allow latecomers to slip into the group with minimal fuss (see below). People are more likely to come on time if a fixed start time is included when you set the ground rules.

From an audience to an interactive group

When your class members first meet, they are a room full of individuals who just happen to be in the same place at the same time. If you want them to become a group, you will have to devote time and energy to getting the process started. Then, during the course, you will need to keep going back to the needs of the group *as a group* to keep it working well.

From the first moment when people start working together as a group, an effective leader has to balance two strands in order for the group to flourish. One strand, 'the task', consists of the work that people have come together to do. In this case, the task is preparing for the birth of a baby and the early weeks of parenthood. The other strand, 'the process', refers to anything that keeps people functioning well *as a group*.

Spending time getting acquainted, or members telling each other about their journey to the class, may seem like a waste of time – 'why not just get on with it? That's why they came!' However, class leaders who plunge straight into work are like house builders who start bricklaying ('the task') without spending time drawing up plans and laying the foundations ('the process'). For a while just laying bricks seems more efficient, but it soon becomes clear that foundations are essential. For bigger, better, more complex houses, scaffolding is also needed alongside bricklaying, each job getting now more and now less attention as seems appropriate.

The same principles hold true for groups. When either the 'task' or the 'group process' is neglected, group members will probably feel frustrated and dissatisfied. Starting the whole business with the group process allows people time to settle and to get to know each other, and lays the foundations for interactive learning.

At first, some people may be reluctant to join in. They may be shy, unsure what to do, suspicious or even contrary. If you treat everyone with gentle respect, give the class members easy, non-threatening things to do and explain exactly what you want of them, they begin to relax and trust both you and each other. After you have started a few groups, you will know that you just have to carry the group's awkwardness until they begin to relate to each other and settle into the work that the group is there to do. It helps everyone if you stay *looking* confident through those early sticky moments. People usually *do* settle, and it is worth it. Working with a group is far more effective and fun than standing in front of a passive audience.

Introductions

In order to feel safe and belong, people need to know each other's names and establish common interests, aims and ways of relating to each other.

The traditional way of starting is to use introductions, generally known icebreakers, in which people are asked to say their name in front of the whole group. Sometimes icebreakers include things like introducing someone else, throwing balls and calling out people's names, or leading people blindfolded around the room The trouble with icebreakers is that they can be counterproductive, because they often raise rather than reduce anxiety.

We suggest that instead of icebreaking, you use an ice-melting process. We believe that this is the single most important step you can take to form a group that will interact, try things out and develop supportive and hopefully long-term relationships. Ice-melters:

- help people to get to know each other gradually, starting in pairs or fours, then joining with another group and another until they have met at least half the class (see below)
- are less stressful because they avoid putting people on the spot
- encourage people to move and to relinquish ownership of their chair. People tend to choose a chair when they arrive and metaphorically spread their beach towel on it, returning to it throughout the course. This means that they are always likely to sit next to the same people and are less likely to get to know everyone, especially in a large class. The key to getting people to relinquish ownership of 'their' chair is to ask them to put their coats and bags outside the circle, rather than hanging them on or leaving them under the chair. In short, if their 'kit is off the chair', they are less likely to keep returning to the same one
- help people establish common interests and concerns and discuss what they have come for
- change the format from an audience with a speaker into an interactive learning group
- *lay an essential foundation for all further interactive learning and group activities.*

Here we describe a three-stage ice-melting process. First introduce yourself and talk for only a few minutes about domestic matters like where the fire escape is, how to find the lavatories, when the coffee breaks will be, and what time the class will end.

Stage one

Ask people to find someone in the room they don't know and give them something very specific and carefully chosen to talk about. Help them to get to know each other gradually. Avoid questions about what they do or where they live, as these can be socially divisive. Ask them to tell each other their names, when their baby is due, and where their baby will be born. You could add another topic – for example, ask them to say one thing about themselves that has nothing whatsoever to do with work or babies that they would be willing to share with the whole group later on;

suggest that they talk about what it was like getting to the class; or, if you intend to establish ground rules, ask them to discuss what should be included.

If you have couples, keep them together and ask them to pair with another couple. Before everyone sits down in their groups, ask them to 'get their kit off the chairs'.

Asking people to pair up always provokes a bit of anxiety. It helps if you:

- acknowledge this – 'this is probably the worst thing I'll ask you to do in the whole course'
- stand up and take centre stage yourself – this encourages other people to move
- make sure that nobody is left standing – gently encourage people who are reluctant, and help them to find a partner. If you have odd numbers, make a threesome (or a group of six if it is a couples' class). Once they are in pairs or fours, repeat the instruction because they will probably have forgotten it while they were concentrating on finding a partner. Alternatively, write the instruction on a flip chart
- give people only a short time in their groups – it is always better to stop people too soon rather than too late. Listen to the noise level in the room, and move on as soon as it starts to drop.

Stage two

Ask each group to join up with another group. Join three groups if you have an odd number.

Once the larger groups are formed, ask them to draw up their chairs in a circle *and take turns to talk*. This is important, as it encourages the quieter ones to have their say and reminds those who tend to dominate to hold back. A nice way of summing up this request is to say, 'nobody speaks twice before everyone has spoken once'. You could ask people to say their names, and when their baby is due. You could add another question, such as 'What's good and what's hard about pregnancy?'. This helps parents to focus on what they have in common, and enables them to share experiences. Choose your words carefully. For example, the word 'pregnancy' includes partners, whereas 'being pregnant' does not.

Stage three

When the noise level drops or people start leaning back and looking less interested, move on and join up the groups. Ideally, you should land up with not more than two groups. If you have an odd number of groups, ask one group to divide back into their original twos or fours and each join a different group.

Again remind class members to take turns, ask them to say their name and when their baby is due, and invite them to set the agenda for the antenatal course. Here are two ways of finding out what parents want:

- Give each group a sheet of flip chart paper and a felt-tip pen and ask them to take turns to say what they want, while one person does the charting. People become more relaxed if you explain that you do not need to know who wants what and that spelling is unimportant. Ask them to make sure that everyone has at least one turn.
- Alternatively, provide each group with a set of agenda-setting cards on which are written a range of topics and issues that they can choose from. The minimum card size for easy reading is A5 with large print. When devising these cards, you need to remember three things:
  a. Use their language.
  b. Choose wording that makes the topic sound interesting and relevant to them. Each card should offer them a carrot (something they want to hear about), not a stick (something you want to tell them).
  c. Use broad headings. This makes it unlikely that the group will exclude things that they really would benefit from hearing about. For example, you could have a card for each aspect of technology and intervention, but this may be very off-putting and could result in class members saying that they don't want to discuss any of them! Instead you could have one card, e.g. *'your baby during labour'*, which would allow you to discuss a whole variety of topics – in this case, the baby's position, moulding, monitoring, acceleration, forceps, Ventouse, and Caesarean birth.

Here are the topics we include on our agenda setting cards. You will see that at nearly half relate to life after birth. This makes it plain that classes are not just about labour. You could also include some blank cards so that parents can add their own topics.

Changes at the end of pregnancy
Pregnancy – looking after yourself
Preparing for birth
When to call the midwife
What are contractions?
Choices about pain relief
Labour – what to expect
If it doesn't go as you hope

Your baby at birth
Welcoming your baby
Leaving your partner and baby in hospital

Easing backache
Sex during pregnancy

How labour starts
The stages of labour
Managing pain in labour
Making choices for labour
The baby during labour
Labour partners – what to expect
What the labour partner can do
Being in hospital
Having your baby at home

Feeding your baby	What new-born babies need
Feelings and reactions after the birth	Taking your baby home
Keeping your baby safe	Sex after birth
The first few weeks after birth	Contraception
After the birth, getting help and support	If your baby is unwell
After the birth, looking after yourself	Baby resuscitation

Once people have completed their agenda sheets or selected their cards, bring the whole group back together again for a name round, followed by a review of the topics they want to cover and, if you include them, a discussion about ground rules. Having talked to at least half the group, most people will be more comfortable about saying their name to the whole group than they would have been at the start of the class. They will also want to find out what topics and issues the other group have chosen.

This whole sequence takes about 25 minutes. Whether or not you wish to spend time in this way will depend on how well you want the group to know each other. If they are only meeting for an hour and will not meet again, foursomes could agree on and list three things they want to do in that time and display their lists on the wall. The whole group could then discuss the lists together. This would take about 25 per cent of your time, but it would be time well spent. Not only would you find out for sure that you were doing what the parents wanted, but they would be in the mood to talk and interact. You can draw on this for the rest of that hour.

On the other hand, if the group is working together for a whole day or is scheduled to meet several times over the next few weeks, you could decide to spend even more than 25 minutes helping everyone to meet, talking, setting an agenda and doing a name round.

If your group is small, you could use a two-stage ice-melter and leave the room for a short time after you have set up each stage. This helps a small group to talk and interact without feeling that they are being observed.

Name rounds

Even if people wear nametags, encourage everyone to say her or his name to the whole group. This lets everyone know how each name is pronounced, and may encourage the quiet ones, having spoken once, to try speaking again. You might want to negotiate with the group as to what form of address will be used. Will everyone – including the teacher – use first names? If you are working with members of minority ethnic groups, check how their naming system works so that you can find out what they would like to be called. You could either do this in advance by consulting a specialist book (see Schott and Henley, 1996), or do it with the group, asking them for help. It is worth spending time on names; a group will work better if everyone knows each other, and people are more likely to form lasting relationships.

Name rounds come in all sorts of styles. Choose non-threatening approaches, otherwise you will undo the good work you achieved through ice-melting. For the first class, you could ask parents to say their name, when their baby is due, and something about themselves. Model this by starting the round off yourself. At the first meeting, keep it light and safe – 'I'm Judy and I'm wearing blue socks', 'I'm Judith and I am not sure what colour to paint my bedroom'.

You may need to repeat name-learning exercises a surprising number of times to help expectant parents learn each other's names. They are often so absorbed in their own worlds, forgetful and anxious, that it takes them longer to fix names in their brains. Groups will welcome a new variant of a name round each time you do it. At subsequent classes you could start by inviting them to say their name followed by something different each week – for example, how they have been during the week; something good that has happened since the last class; anything they have thought about since the last class; or how their baby has been during the last week.

Towards the end of the course, when people are relaxed and comfortable with each other, you could ask them to say their name and something about it. Make sure you say that they can choose how much or how little to say. For example, they could simply say 'My name is Judith'. This is important, because not everyone wants to talk about their name and not everyone knows, for example, who chose their name or why. It is also important to ask everyone to listen with complete respect and without comment. As a society we are not very respectful of people's names – we shorten them, lengthen them and tease people about them. This is unhelpful, since most people are sensitive about their name, whether they like it or not.

When you are leading a round of any sort, start with yourself to set the tone, then turn towards each person in turn and give him or her your complete attention as they speak. When people have finished, you could nod, smile or thank them. This acknowledges the speaker and lets the next person know it is his or her turn. If you set up a round, it is important that you do not let anyone interrupt it. Stories and discussion can wait until everyone has had equal time.

Setting ground rules

All groups develop patterns of interacting, even if they do not realize it. You may want to agree some ground rules with your group so that everyone can share responsibility for maintaining them. You may wish to propose a few rules yourself; write them down and ask people to discuss them during the ice-melting process. Afterwards, ask for additions and changes before agreeing and displaying them for all to see. Here are some we use.

Confidentiality
By this, we mean not only that people agree that what is said or done in this group stays in the room, but also that what people say or do in small groups stays in the groups. People are often willing to say things in groups of three or four that they would be horrified to hear repeated in a group of 16. This restriction includes prompting along the lines of 'that's like what you were saying, Zoe, when we talked about ...'.

Equal time
Suggest that members pay attention to how often and how long they speak. This helps the talkers hold back and listen. Given time and space, the more reluctant people will offer their ideas and experiences. By agreeing to share time more or less equally the whole group takes responsibility for this, although they will need frequent prompts in the early sessions lest the dominant people fall back on old habits.

Listening with respect
We all find it easier to listen to those we agree with than to those with whom we disagree. By suggesting that people listen as hard to the differences between them as to the similarities, you help them feel freer to speak and encourage those who are firmly fixed in any one notion to begin to explore other ways of thinking and feeling. This is especially important in relation to pregnancy and birth, where few issues have a clear right or wrong answer yet most have passionate advocates – class leaders too! You can model respect yourself by including everyone, even if you disagree with what they say or do. This will probably mean that you will need to examine your own feelings and attitudes from time to time.

Setting a course agenda

You are as unlikely to start a course without a plan as you are to start a long journey without a map and itinerary. Unlike most of your group you have 'travelled' this way before, so you are likely to know the topics and activities that usually are relevant and useful. However, your knowledge and experience must be tailored to suit each group. Since you are not a mind reader, the only way to find out about people's needs and priorities is to ask them. We have described two methods of agenda setting above. There is a third method, which can be used in addition to either agenda sheets or agenda-setting cards.

The safe pot
Because people are often reluctant to mention things that really concern or frighten them, it is helpful to offer them a way to raise these issues anonymously. Place a container, the 'safe pot', and paper and pencils somewhere unobtrusive so that people can use them without being the centre of attention. Invite people to write down (at any time throughout

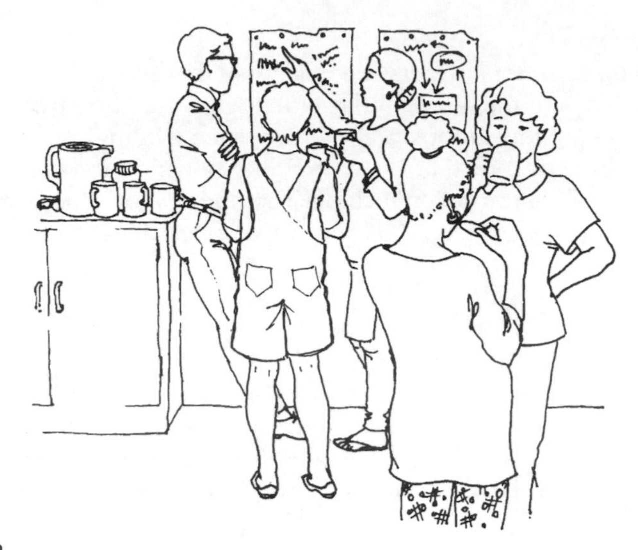

Figure 5.2

the course) topics they would like covered in the course, including the things that most worry them. Stress that there is no need to give their names or say which is their topic. Ask them to place their papers in the safe pot.

At the end of each class you can check what has appeared in the pot, and ensure that you cover it before the end of the course. Remove the pot before the last class to avoid being inundated with topics with no time to cover them! We suggest that you do not ask participants to draw topics out of the pot and read them out to the class. Think how you might feel as a participant, if you were expected to read out 'stillbirth'!

Responding to their needs

Implicit in any agenda-planning exercise is your commitment to adapt what you do to accommodate participants' wishes. You not only have to do it, you have to be *seen* to do it. Start by reviewing their requests. If they have written agenda sheets, review their requests by displaying them and going through them so that you can clarify exactly what they want. If you used cards, you could ask each group to lay out their choices on the floor and invite people to go and see what the other group has chosen.

You then need to turn the sheets or cards into a manageable agenda. One way is to list all the things they want on one sheet of flip-chart paper. This can be kept for the life of the group and displayed at each class (Figure 5.2). At the end of each class, ask the group to tell you what can be ticked off. In this way you both demonstrate that you are responding to their requests, and let them decide when their needs have been met.

If there are too many topics to cover in the time you have, you can ask the group to prioritize. A quick and efficient way of doing this is to ask the class to vote for the topics they most want to cover. Decide first how many topics you have time for. For example, if you have four topics left to cover and time for only two, tell everyone that they each have two votes and ask them to decide which two topics they most want to cover. Ask for a show of hands for each topic, count up the votes, and then tackle the topics in the order of priority set by the group.

Forming small groups

As well as forming different sized groups for ice-melting, you can form groups of different sizes for different tasks throughout the course. This enables people to meet and talk to most if not all the other participants, and helps to keep people alert and involved. Groups of more than 14 people tend to function like an audience – some people will contribute while others tend to keep quiet. Therefore, the larger the class the more important small group work becomes.

Matching size to task

In general, people are more likely to feel safe to talk openly in twos, or in groups of three or four. So if you invite people to talk about emotive topics or what they think and feel, form groups of two or a maximum of four. Groups of this size are also good for enabling quieter people to talk. People in groups of five or six can share experiences, especially if they have already practised listening to each other in groups of two or three. You need six to ten people if you want them to generate ideas or make lists. Smaller groups of people may not have enough information between them to complete a task that requires a certain amount of knowledge. You will find suggestions for appropriate group sizes for different activities throughout the book.

Dividing the class

You can form several different group sizes out of most classes. For example, if you have 24 people you could form:

- twelve groups of two
- eight groups of three
- six groups of four
- four groups of six
- three groups of eight
- two groups of twelve.

You can use this approach to divide groups of 12, 30 or even 50, although some groups do not divide so neatly! If you have uneven numbers, work out how to include everyone – 'we'll have six groups of two and one group of three'. Always make sure that nobody has the embarrassment of being the odd one out. If you teach couples, keep partners together at least until the group is well established.

There are many different ways to form different sized groups. By using a variety of methods, you can ensure that people mix and keep them entertained at the same time. Here are some approaches that we use:

- *In twos*. Check you have an even number, and ask people to pair up with the person next to them, or with someone they have not spoken to yet.
- *In fours*. Join two pairs that have already worked together. In a couples' class, ask each couple to pair with another. Alternatively you could go round the group allocating a number to each woman (or couple) – one, two, three, four – or use a variation such as orange, apple, pear, banana; or north, south, east, west. You could also divide people according to the months of their birth – 'hands up if your birthday is in January to March'. This is not so reliable and you may have to adjust the groups to get them roughly the same size, but it is fun and often gets people talking about birthdays and star signs. You can adapt all these methods to form groups of three, five and six. If you teach couples you can use birthdays twice, dividing couples up one week on the basis of her birthday and the following week on the basis of her partner's. This will result in different combinations of people.
- *In half*. You could: draw an 'equator' through the middle of the group, but vary the line each time you use this method. You could number one, two, one, two round the group, or use a variation such as eggs, bacon, eggs, bacon. In a group of 20 or more, try asking people to fold their arms and see if the right or their left arm is on top; or you can ask them to clasp their hands and interlace their fingers and see if their left or right thumb is on top. These methods are likely to give you two similar sized groups, but do not work well if you have less than 20 class members. If you teach couples, you can use each of the last two methods twice in the course (see using birthdays, above).
- *Common interest groups*. You can also group people who have things in common (see Chapter 17) and, later in the group, form single sex groups (see Chapter 13). This gives people an opportunity to talk about their particular needs and perspectives with people who are in the same boat.

Whenever you form small groups it helps to:

- Ensure, before anyone moves, that they have remembered which group

they are in. You could say something like 'would all the apples raise their hand please?'.
- Allocate each group a specific area of the room, and make sure everyone knows where to go.
- Explain clearly what you want them to do, once the groups are formed.

Key points

- People bring preconceived expectations, hopes and anxieties with them to the first class.
- Effective classes take into account people's needs for safety, security, comfort and a sense of belonging.
- First impressions have lasting effects.
- The ideal venue seldom exists. It is important to give time and thought to arranging the room you have to its best advantage.
- Good directions and signposting reduce anxiety and frustration.
- A warm welcome helps to reduce anxiety and sets a positive and constructive tone.
- Ice-melters enable people to get to know each other, and are an important foundation for interactive learning.
- Establishing the parents' agenda is an essential first step to meeting their needs.
- Using small group work and dividing people in different ways maintains interest and ensures that class members mingle.

References

Schott, J. and Henley, A. (1996). *Culture, Religion and Childbearing in a Multiracial Society: A Handbook for Health Professionals*, Chapter 14. Butterworth-Heinemann.

Chapter 6

Giving information

This chapter discusses the role and scope of information giving in antenatal classes. It offers practical suggestions that can help parents remember and use what they have heard.

Traditionally, giving information has occupied most of each class. The leader holds the floor for long periods, while the parents sit and listen – or sometimes just sit! Ironically, neither is usually enthusiastic about this approach. Class leaders often dread being the sole focus of attention, may long for more participation and feedback, and are genuinely dismayed to discover how little participants can remember and apply. Some parents will be satisfied, but many feel bored or frustrated. Later on, when they realize that passive listening has not equipped them to cope with labour or early parenthood, they may feel let down.

The question that most class leaders struggle with is 'How much information can I pack in to ensure that I cover everything?'. We suggest that you try replacing this question with 'How much information can parents absorb in the time available?'. An information-laden course might appear to meet parents' needs, but if they cannot retain or use what they have heard, nothing has actually been achieved. This means it is essential to consider how much information to give, and for how long people can listen at any one time and absorb what they hear.

The average human attention span is around 20 minutes (see Chapter 3). Pregnancy shortens even this brief span, because anxiety and tiredness interfere with active listening. Pregnancy amnesia also reduces women's ability to retain information (Sharp *et al.*, 1993). If attention levels are limited, it makes sense to shorten lectures. We suggest that you aim to talk for a maximum of five minutes at a time.

The five-minute lecture and how to give it

If you give lectures, you owe it to yourself and your listeners to be really effective. The following key points can help.

Keep it short

As a rule of thumb, never talk for longer than five minutes at a time. Parents often seem to listen for much longer than this. They are often so hungry for information and so anxious to 'get things right' that they will sit quietly for a long time, but they may not actually be learning anything.

Cover large topics in small sections

If you consider the mass of information required to cover labour or pain relief, it makes sense to break each topic down into smaller, more digestible, bite-sized chunks. When you are planning what to say, start by taking the topic apart. For instance, you can treat labour as a story with many 'chapters' – how labour starts, the changeover to active labour, early first stage, late first stage and so on. You can describe each of these in a five-minute lecture with time between each for a linked activity – discussion, relaxation, or appropriate positions for that stage of labour (Schott, 1995).

You can cover any large topic in this way. For example, you can intersperse information on the different forms of pharmacological pain relief with reflection in small groups, or with self-help pain management techniques such as massage.

If you give good information in five-minute chunks, you might spend a total of 45 minutes of a two-hour session talking to your listening group. This gives you time to intersperse your lectures with active learning, relevant physical skills, discussion, reflection and invitations to ask further questions. All of these activities can enhance and build on the information you have given. Handling information in this way does not necessarily reduce the *total* amount of information you give, but does change the way in which you do it.

Identify essential information

> *. . . most courses are over- rather than under-loaded. Perhaps the reasons for this is that the teachers tend to take themselves and their own range of knowledge as the norm for their students.*
>
> (Rogers, 2000)

When we introduce the concept of the five-minute lecture to class leaders, some balk at the idea. There is so much to say, and it all seems important. It can be hard to leave things out – after all, pregnancy, birth and new parenthood are the things around which your working life revolves. It would be surprising if you didn't find them fascinating and want to share your insights and experience with others. However, limited time, limited attention spans and the sheer impossibility of telling the group everything force cuts on you. 'If you try to say too much, you end up saying nothing' (Strong, 1996).

You could probably give ten or more pieces of information that you could offer about any given topic, but most people will remember only a few. What people remember tends to be the dramatic rather than the things that might be really useful to them. Advertisers, who are experts in effective communication, sum up what they want people to hear in one succinct message (Strong, 1996). We suggest that you tell people a maximum of three things that are factual and will improve their ability to deal with the actual experience.

This means being highly selective and deciding on three basic facts about each topic. One way to sort out the essential from the fascinating but optional is to imagine this scene. You are at an airport and your transatlantic flight is about to be called. You are making a long-distance telephone call from the airport to a close friend who is eight and a half months pregnant. Just as your flight is announced, your friend says, 'Tell me about breastfeeding'. You only have time for three short sentences. Imagine she will not have any other sources of information or support. What do you say?

You could probably talk quite eloquently about the anatomy of the breast, the physiology, the let-down reflex, colostrum, foremilk, hindmilk and so on. But however interesting, this information it is unlikely to enable a woman to establish breastfeeding. To breastfeed, she must know how to position the baby, how to recognize a good latch, and the law of demand and supply. Without these three, breastfeeding won't work. Of course there is more to it – whole libraries of books have been written on breastfeeding! But what does she have to know to get started?

Exactly the same scenario will help you decide the three (or four) points that are essential about any topic. What are the three essential things about second stage? About contractions? About postnatal depression? About vitamin K? About what newborn babies need? Stick to facts. Giving personal opinions or telling them your feelings about a topic is nearly always unhelpful. Facts, on the other hand, are of concrete use. Where relevant, include information about what women and their partners might feel as well as what might happen. This helps parents to prepare for the actual experience.

Some health professionals are concerned that this approach it might leave them open to criticism from parents later – 'you never told us about . . .'. In fact comments or complaints of this sort are just as likely if your classes are stuffed with information, since people cannot possibly remember it all. A few health professionals worry about litigation – 'we've got to tell them everything or they might sue'. This assumes that classes are an extension of clinical care rather than a forum for education. Antenatal classes can never be a substitute for good communication or for obtaining informed consent during clinical care.

Three things three times

You can increase the chances that your listeners will hear and absorb the three things that you have decided to say if you:

- tell them what you are going to say. For example, 'I want to talk about what women say about having forceps; about how you can help yourself; and about the things that might help you afterwards . . .'.
- give the information. For example, offer a sentence quoting what women say about forceps, and a sentence quoting a man's experience. Then offer two suggestions for coping with forceps during the birth, each no more than a couple of sentences long. Then suggest one or two ways of keeping comfortable and speeding recovery.
- End by summarizing the key points again, using different words.

Lectures are a useful way of transmitting information. However, people can only remember a limited amount, and lectures do not necessarily promote reflection or understanding; nor are they an effective way of changing attitudes or developing skills (Bligh, 1998).

The Chinese have a proverb: I hear and I forget – I see and I remember – I do and I understand. If you vary your approach by using teaching aids and interspersing your five-minute lectures with small group discussions, or activities that enable people to use the information you have given, your message becomes more memorable (see Chapters 8 and 9).

Delivering information in this way takes a bit of practice. You could try out your first efforts on a friend or a small group of supportive colleagues.

Language

Health professionals often do not realize that they speak their own unique language – NHS. In fact, each speaks the particular dialect of their profession. The phrases and acronyms used by midwives, obstetricians, physiotherapists and health visitors are very different. Not only do these dialects provide short cuts when communicating with each other, they also demonstrate professional credibility. They are assiduously learned until they become an automatic and almost unconscious part of speech patterns at work.

The language of professional textbooks compounds the problem. The style is often complex, technical and usually objective. This approach subtly implies that what is being described is separate not only from the author's own experience but also from that of the reader. Here is an example from a book written for parents and described as being 'in straightforward, non-technical language':

The pelvic floor consists of a layer of muscle and fibrous tissue that extends across the lower part of the bony pelvis from the lower edge of the symphysis pubis to the tip of the sacrum.

(Bourne, 1989)

You would never guess from reading this sentence that both the author and the reader are sitting on pelvic floors of their own!

Many parents find professional language exclusive, confusing or even alienating. Whatever you talk about – anatomy, technology, feelings or experiences – you are dealing with issues that intimately affect the people you are talking to. A woman hears 'she's effaced', and wonders what her face has to do with giving birth. Parents hearing 'cephalic' might think that there is something wrong with their baby. Midwives say 'she's fully' – a statement that parents are likely to find baffling, especially as it is sometimes unconsciously accompanied by a two-fingered gesture, indicating the degree of dilatation. At worst, inappropriate language can cause devastation. A midwife told us of a woman who was extremely distressed because she had heard a doctor say that she had a 'monkey's arse'. What he had actually said was 'a multips os'.

This does not mean that you should not use anatomically correct terms and professional phrases. Parents are bound to hear some of these, and most would prefer to understand them. When parents know technical terms, they often feel more empowered and in control. Not only can they ask questions and understand the answers, they also elicit different behaviour from the health professionals they meet. 'How far has my cervix dilated?' prompts a different answer to 'Is it opening up?'.

We have found that linking lay terms with professional language works well. It helps to ensure that everyone understands you and reduces the risk of patronizing people by oversimplifying or baffling them with technicalities. Many medical terms have a familiar equivalent that will convey the meaning equally well. Pain relief does not mean exactly the same as analgesia, or bleeding the same as haemorrhage, but each is a more than adequate substitute. So, for example, you could say: the uterus or womb; the cervix or neck of the womb; the waters, amniotic fluid or liquor; the placenta or afterbirth; back passage or rectum; vagina or birth canal.

As well as finding ways of describing medical procedures and translating medical terms, you need to decide what language to use when talking about intimate human activities such as sex and excretion. We have been taught to be embarrassed about these subjects, and they are often referred to rather indirectly, coyly, in a jokey way, or not at all. Some health professionals use rather formal terms and expressions, which can sound stilted and may well not be understood. Others use euphemisms, and a few use more graphic terms commonly referred to as four-letter words.

- What words will you use to talk about sex? Will you use anatomical terms? Will you talk about making love, sexual intercourse, penetrative

sex, having sex, or use one of the many euphemisms that abound? What words will you use for male and female sex organs?
- What words will you use when talking about excretion? Going to the toilet/loo? Passing water/urine? Having a pee/doing a wee? Having a motion/opening your bowels?

It is vital to use words you are comfortable with, otherwise you will just convey embarrassment or tension. However, it is also vital to be precise so that people know exactly what you mean. For example, making love is a broader and vaguer term than penetrative sex. As well as identifying words that you can use freely, you need to think about the people in your classes. What words will they understand and be able to relate to? Finding the right pitch takes practice and means observing the responses you get. It may also mean that you have to adapt your language and your attitudes! If you find some words difficult, practise saying them out loud in private. Then say them out loud in front of a mirror. You may decide some words are not for you, and that is fine. However, they may be right for others. It is important to be open-minded and flexible so that you can remain relaxed if someone in your class uses words that you would not use yourself.

Make it personal

Whether you are talking about anatomy, technology, feelings or experiences, you are dealing with issues that intimately affect the people you are talking with – either things that are actually present in the room, or that are anticipated as possible experiences in the near future.

Talk directly to parents instead of using the third person ('you' rather than 'she' or 'a pregnant woman'). This helps people to connect what you are saying to themselves. 'The baby' becomes 'your baby'. However, take care. If you use 'you' or 'your', it needs to apply to *every single person* in the room. 'Your baby' excludes anyone expecting twins, and 'your labour' excludes women anticipating a Caesarean. These differences need to be acknowledged regularly. For example, you may need to make a special effort to say 'your baby or your babies' or ' labour, or however your baby is born'.

You need to take even more care with the words 'you' and 'your' when partners are present. 'Your baby' includes everyone; 'pressure on your back passage' does not. Even the occasional use of 'you' or 'your' that excludes the partners will cancel out all your assertions about this class being for them too. To avoid this, try directing your comments to the women first and then to the partners. For example: 'at this stage women often feel pressure on their back passage. Her partner often notices that she catches her breath and seems to want to push at the height of a contraction'.

Reflect the parents' point of view

Try to reflect the parents' point of view in the words you use. A 'delivery' describes the experience of midwives and doctors; parents and babies experience 'a birth'. Hospitals 'discharge' people, but parents 'go home'. How would you describe 'hospital admission' in parent-centred language?

It is sometimes more difficult to stand in parents' shoes when describing topics or giving information. For example, when we ask a group of health professionals to describe the feelings and experiences of the second stage of labour, the most common things they mention are time limits, the various movements of the baby, and crowning. They also mention the feelings generated by waiting for the baby's birth, excitement at first sighting the head, and the hard work involved for mothers and their helpers. When we ask mothers, very different things emerge. Some mention the same things as professionals, but most describe feelings of stretching and burning, the frustration of two steps forward and one step back pushing, feeling stuck and desperate, and pain. When you talk about the second stage, whose experience are you describing – yours, the partner's, the mother's, the baby's? All four are valid, but only the last three are helpful to your group.

Using analogies

Comparisons are commonly used to describe the unfamiliar. People who have pain are asked if it is stabbing, throbbing, burning, sharp or dull. The taste and bouquet of wine are described by comparing them to familiar smells and tastes. Carefully chosen analogies are especially useful in antenatal classes because they clarify the unknown. If you are trying to explain a physiological process, or talking about a complex or potentially scary topic, try comparing it with something familiar. Make sure your images are constructive and positive. Comparisons between stitches and 'sitting on barbed wire', or giving birth and defecation, are likely to be more shocking than helpful. Here are some examples to stimulate your creative thinking.

- The placenta is the most efficient room service in the world.
- Babies are like barometers. They sense the atmosphere around them.
- Forceps are a bit like metal salad servers. They come in two halves, and fit together to cradle the baby's head.
- Labour can feel like running a marathon.
- The way the baby's head changes direction when it reaches the mother's pelvic floor muscles is a bit like the way your foot changes direction when putting on a Wellington boot. At first your foot travels straight down. When your toes reach the bottom, your foot changes direction in order to move forward.

- Your circulation is a bit like a child's swimming ring. Imagine blowing up the ring to a pressure of, say, 80. Now imagine squeezing one side of the ring. The pressure will go up, say to 120. When you let go, it goes back to 80. Exactly the same thing happens to your blood pressure. When your heart contracts the pressure goes up, and in between each heartbeat the pressure drops to the lower level. This is why, when we measure blood pressure, there are two different levels.
- Having an epidural caesarean can feel like someone doing the washing up in your tummy.
- Carrying active twins can feel like a boxful of puppies.
- A fast labour can feel like being in a spin drier.
- After the birth, a woman's tummy looks a bit like a half-set jelly.

Perhaps the most fruitful use of metaphor comes when describing the inevitability and accelerating pattern of labour contractions. Here are some examples that parents have offered us over the years:

- '... like standing up to my knees in water and seeing the waves coming then crashing over me then fading out up on the beach.'
- '... like a roller-coaster ride, with the big bit getting higher all the time.'
- '... like letting go at the top of a helter-skelter ... you go faster and faster, and just have to keep going till you reach the end.'

Catchy phrases

Catchy phrases are useful because they are memorable and often fun. They sum up complex information in a succinct package. Companies pay advertising agencies a fortune for them, and celebrities who have a personal catchphrase win rounds of applause each time they repeat it. Here are a few examples, some in common use, to help you start thinking of some of your own:

- to convey the concept of demand and supply – 'sucking makes milk'
- for fathers worried about the onset of labour – 'if she's wondering if she's in labour, she's not'
- to sum up breathing for labour or for any stressful situation – 'if in doubt, breathe out'
- as a reminder about the onset of labour – 'if your waters go, please let us know'
- for positioning at the breast – 'chest to chest and chin to breast'
- for labour (and to a certain extent for early parenting) – 'just let go and go with the flow'
- for infant sleeping and cot death prevention – 'feet to foot and back to sleep' (to prevent or relieve calf cramp – 'stretch your leg with toes to nose'.

The effects of individual words

Euphemisms are unhelpful. Saying 'discomfort' when you really mean 'pain', or glossing over the mechanics of how a scalp electrode is attached, leaves parents less prepared for these events than if you say nothing at all (see Chapter 14). You can be truthful without choosing the starkest words or the most negative slant on things. A scalp electrode may indeed be 'screwed into' the baby's head, but a less emotive phrase like 'clipped onto' will do just as well. Some words just sound more painful, like 'cut' (rather than 'snip') to describe an episiotomy. The tricky bit is finding the middle way where truth and sensitivity meet. This is a balancing act that takes constant monitoring.

Developing accurate, realistic descriptions

Class leaders often need to describe objects, events and feelings that are either outside parents' experiences or inside the mother's body. Of course visual aids like photographs or actual objects can help, but you will still be called upon to conjure up a realistic picture of things that are mysterious or hidden. It can take time to develop a repertoire of suitable descriptions and word pictures. Here's a pattern that works for us.

- *What is it?* One sentence is almost always enough if you think hard about what you want to describe. Waffle confuses and irritates the listeners and can give the impression that either you do not really want them to understand or you are unsure about what you should say.
- *How will it feel?* Objective information does not prepare people for the subjective experience (Niven, 1992). Realistic information includes sensory descriptions – what the mother might feel, see, hear, touch, smell or taste. Include as many of the five senses as you can. If partners are present, use the same approach to describe what they might experience. Don't forget the baby – what will he or she experience? The more vivid and accurate your descriptions are, the more real they will be. Again, keep it short and never use three words when one will do. For example, when discussing forceps, you could tell parents about the different kinds of forceps and offer details about how they are applied. Whilst those applying the forceps certainly need to know about the different types and their uses, expectant parents might find it more useful if you talk about the 'clang' forceps produce when picked up, what the partner will see, the various sensations mothers describe when forceps are inserted and traction is applied, or what effects forceps might have on the baby's experience of birth.
- *What will everyone involved be doing?* If it will increase parents' understanding, describe briefly what one or two other people in the room will be doing, but only after you have described what the parents might see, hear and feel. For example, once you have described what the parents

might experience, you could say: 'Forceps are always done by a doctor, and he or she may have to pull quite hard to ease the baby out as the mother pushes', or 'If you have a Caesarean, a paediatrician will be there waiting to check the baby when he or she is born'. You can follow this pattern for almost everything you are called upon to describe. How would you use these pointers to describe an epidural Caesarean? A Ventouse extraction? An episiotomy?

Other ways of giving information

Discussion and questions

Discussion often provides lots of information and ideas, both for other group members and for the leader. Small group discussion is especially useful, as it provides safety for people to explore their own thinking and formulate their own comments and questions. You can use it to focus people's attention on a topic you are about to cover – for example, instead of launching into a lecture on the onset of labour, you could form small groups and ask them to talk about how they feel about going into labour. Small group discussion after a five-minute lecture can provide you with feedback, and guidance about else this group wants to know. This enables you to tailor the amount of information to the group needs (see Chapter 7).

Handouts

Handouts can be a very useful adjunct, and can seem like an easy way to convey a lot of information. However, successful handouts and leaflets require considerable thought and planning. If you use or intend to use handouts, you may find it useful to reflect on the following.

- How much written material is given routinely to each woman during her entire pregnancy? In some areas it amounts to a mini paper mountain. Try collecting a copy of everything that is used where you work, and measure the pile. Is it all really necessary? Do some of the handouts duplicate information? Are most people likely to read them all?
- Are your handouts written in plain English, with short, clear sentences?
- Are the style and layout attractive and uncluttered?
- Is the content practical, up to date and, where relevant, research-based?
- Is the message a carrot or a stick?
- Do any illustrations and text reflect the cultures and lifestyles of the people in your area?
- Are your handouts available in the languages spoken by people in your area?

Starting with what they know

This chapter has concentrated on how to provide parents with information. However, parents do not come to antenatal classes as empty vessels waiting to be filled; most will have heard a great deal about pregnancy, birth and parenthood. For example, news coverage of pregnancy and parent-related issues is becoming ever more frequent. Pain relief is regularly covered by popular pregnancy magazines, and everyone will have heard stories about how labour starts. In most groups the more academic members will have read several books, and increasingly people are surfing the net.

By starting with what parents already know, you demonstrate respect for them and can tailor your information to the needs of that group of parents. You may also gain an insight into any inaccuracies or misconceptions that they might have. This gives you a chance to reshape your information to give a more accurate and realistic picture (see Chapter 9).

Key points

- Information giving tends to dominate most antenatal classes, leaving little time for other approaches.
- Instead of concentrating on 'how much information can we pack into the course?', focus on 'how much are parents likely to remember?'
- Peoples' attention span is limited, so it makes sense break up topics into digestible chunks and to use five-minute lectures.
- If people are only likely to remember three things about each topic, tell them three things that will actually be useful to them.
- Linking everyday language to professional terms increases understanding and reduces the chances of parents feeling either baffled or patronized.
- Analogies and catchy phrases increase understanding, are memorable and can be fun.
- Lectures can transfer information, but they do not necessarily promote reflection or understanding.
- People are more likely to understand and remember what they hear if you intersperse five-minute lectures with a range of other activities.

References

Bligh, D. (1998). *What's the Use of Lectures?*, 3rd edn, p. 23. Intellect.
Bourne, G. (1989). *Pregnancy*, p. 38. Cassell Publishers.
Niven, C. (1992). *Psychological Care for Families, Before, During and After Birth*, pp. 63–5. Butterworth-Heinemann.
Rogers, A. (2000). *Teaching Adults*, p. 135. Open University Press.

Schott, J. (1995). Cancel the labour talk. *British Journal of Midwifery*, **3**(10), 517–18.

Sharp, K., Brindle, P. M., Brown, M. W. and Turner, G. (1993). Memory loss during pregnancy. *British Journal of Obstetrics and Gynaecology*, **100**(3), 209–15.

Strong, T. (1996). Tennis balls and prostitutes. What can health care learn from advertising? *King's Fund News*, **19**(3), 4.

Chapter 7

Leading discussion

This chapter outlines the role of discussion in antenatal classes, and offers practical suggestions for initiating, maintaining and ending discussions.

Why include discussion?

Discussions offer benefits that cannot be achieved in any other ways, and are particularly suitable for adults who have wide range of experiences, facts and beliefs to draw upon. Studies have consistently shown that discussion is more likely than lectures to keep people alert, attentive and thoughtful (Bligh, 1998). Many people find it easier to learn and change if they have opportunities to reflect and evaluate what they have heard. If people sit and listen week after week, ask a few questions and then go home with their thoughts locked inside them, they often feel frustrated and even angry. Discussion helps people to express what they think or feel, acknowledge shared problems or beliefs, and formulate questions. Through discussion, they may also discover their own solutions:

> *How do I know what I think till I hear what I say?*
>
> (Source unknown)

Starting with yourself

While many class leaders welcome discussion, some worry about losing control – the discussion might never get started, it will take up too much time, it might get out of hand, or topics might be raised that would be hard to handle. Taking time to explore your feelings about discussion can help you to identify the skills you already have and those that you could develop. How do you feel about:

- participating in a discussion?
- leading a discussion?

- dealing with what might come up?
- setting up small groups that do not involve you?
- starting and ending discussions?

Practical approaches

The following suggestions will either remind you of things you already do or of things you could do. They may need to be adapted and changed to fit your own style and the needs of the particular group you are working with.

Creating safety

A class that is an audience rather than an interactive learning group is unlikely to switch willingly to discussion. You need to lay the foundations from the very first class so that everyone in the group is accustomed interacting with other participants (see Chapter 5). People also need to know in advance what will happen after the discussion. For example, will there be feedback to the whole group? If you are gathering ideas and information, feedback is clearly important. However, if you are using small groups to help people explore their feelings, feedback may be unnecessary and even inhibiting. People may be reluctant to open up if there is a chance that their views or feelings might be fed back to the whole class, especially by someone else. So tell people in advance what will happen afterwards.

Clarifying your purpose and organizing appropriate-sized groupings

The size of the group needs to be tailored to your aim. You need larger groups if you want people to generate information and ideas, and smaller groups if you want them to talk about what they think or feel.

If you want parents to reflect on what they have heard, to say how they feel or to generate questions, you need groups of two, three (or, in a couples' class, a maximum of four). This gives everyone time to talk, and provides enough safety for most people to feel able to contribute. Formal feedback is not usually necessary, since the work is done within the groups. However, you could ask if anyone has comments or questions. In this case, it is essential to make it clear at the outset that participants should only comment or ask about what they themselves think or want to know. Nobody should comment on or repeat anything that another person in the small group has said.

An ideal group size for generating ideas and information is between six and ten people. Fewer than six have only a small range of experiences and ideas to draw on, and they are more likely to get stuck or polarized between widely differing views. More than ten often have too much information and variety to keep track of easily. Participants may feel overwhelmed or confused, and usually a few people dominate or form breakaway subgroups. You can reduce the chances of anyone dominating a group by suggesting that everyone has a turn to speak once before anyone speaks twice. If you want to generate ideas or information, tell people at the start that you will asking for feedback later. Alternatively, give them paper and felt-tip pens so that they can list their ideas.

Encouraging the habit of speech

Being part of an audience and listening for any length of time makes people lose the urge to speak. Frequent short breaks for small group discussion help to keep people involved and alert, and increase their willingness to speak out.

Small group discussion is particularly useful if you want to generate comments and questions. Most leaders have attempted to involve people or tried to get themselves out of a tight corner or break an awkward silence by asking brightly, 'Any questions?'. If you have tried this you will probably have been met, as we have, with total silence, so that your already faltering confidence evaporates completely. Next time you are tempted to ask the whole group for questions, stop! Instead, try forming small groups and asking them to talk about what they think or feel about the topic in hand. This gives you a few minutes to recover your composure, and gives them a chance to let off steam, clarify their thoughts and perhaps formulate questions. You can then ask, 'Are there any comments or questions – before we move on?'. This last phrase allows you to change tack quickly and avoid another awkward silence if nobody responds to your invitation.

Starting a discussion

When you start a discussion you are *inviting* the group to join in, so the warmer your invitation, the more likely they are to respond. They will judge your offer both by the words you say and by the way you say them. Non-verbal messages include:

- *Posture*. Do you lean forward slightly, with a relaxed and open posture, turning your body to face different people in the group – including those to your immediate left and right?
- *Eye contact*. Do your eyes roam the group, making and breaking eye contact with many members, ready to catch the eye of someone willing to respond?
- *Tone of voice*. When you ask a question, does your voice sound questioning and genuinely interested in the response? Do you ask questions slowly, with enough pauses between phrases to allow people to take the question in and understand what you are asking?

- *Silences*. Do you give participants time to respond? If the gap between your question and the first word from them bothers you, try counting to 20 – silently and slowly – while you continue to offer general eye contact and an inviting expression. That may keep you busy while they gather themselves to speak.

Choosing your questions

Think carefully about the questions you use to start a discussion. Only certain types of questions are effective.

Closed questions

These usually have a right or a wrong answer, or invite a 'yes' or a 'no' response. The person asking the question often knows in advance what the answer is likely to be. Closed questions have very little place in antenatal classes, and are no use for starting discussion. Consider, for example, these three questions:

'Who can tell me the three ways that labour starts?'

'What do you know about pain relief, then?'

'What's the best thing to do when a baby cries?'

Some leaders may see such questions as encouraging, and offer them with all the inviting non-verbal cues described above. In fact, they put parents on the spot and expose them to the possibility of feeling silly and showing their ignorance in public. Some parents won't mind and may even welcome the chance to demonstrate their knowledge, sometimes at great length. These are the ones who do not need encouragement. Other parents, however, will be extremely wary, because they remember similar traps from their school days. These are usually the people you would most like to encourage.

Leading questions

These include questions that express your prejudices (e.g. 'Is anyone here really going to bottle feed?') and questions that give participants a clear indication of the answer you want by the way you ask it (e.g. 'So what do you think about manufacturers making vast profits from selling tiny-sized baby clothes that are outgrown after the first two weeks?'). Neither of these approaches is helpful.

Open questions

These are the most effective questions for triggering discussion. Your question will probably be 'open' if:

- it cannot be answered with 'yes' or 'no'

- it has more than one answer
- you have no idea what the answer might be
- it invites people to say as much or as little as they wish.

Open questions need planning and practice. Think first about what you hope the discussion will achieve, and then tailor your questions to fit your aim. Make sure that your questions are relevant to everyone in the room, including partners, and use inclusive language (see Chapters 13 and 17).

If you want parents to explore their attitudes and feelings, try questions like:

> 'What are you most looking forward to?'
>
> 'What thoughts and images flashed through your mind at the first scan?'
>
> 'Which bits about hospital will you find the hardest?'
>
> 'How do you think your baby would like to be welcomed?'
>
> 'What do you think will be good and what will be hard about being a parent?'

If you want parents to talk about whatever is important for them in a particular topic, try questions like:

> 'Suppose you met someone who was trying to get pregnant and she asked, "What are the first three months like?" – what would you definitely mention?'
>
> 'Some women are sure they want drugs for pain relief and some are just as sure they don't. What do you think?'

If you want to encourage them to develop their own strategies and solutions, try questions like:

> 'When you have had a similar problem in the past, what have you tried that might work here, too?'
>
> 'How do you think you might feel about breastfeeding in front of friends and relatives, or in public? Are there people you would feel comfortable about? Are there any with whom you might feel uncomfortable? How could you deal with this?'
>
> 'Three people have mentioned in-laws visiting in the first few days. How do you feel, and what might work best for you and your family?'

Check that the questions you ask link with their own experiences. Asking first-time parents 'How will you cope in the first few days?' will draw blank looks, but you might get them going by asking 'What have you heard people say about the first few days with a new baby?'.

Timing

To be effective, your questions should match the level of comfort and intimacy achieved by the group. Early in a group's life, early in a particular session, or even throughout the life of an open group (where members come and go week by week), some topics may be too hot to handle and the group will either refuse to discuss them or be left feeling threatened and unhappy. These topics are discussed in greater detail in Chapter 14.

However, people may be willing to tackle cooler issues like the physical changes they have noticed in early pregnancy, what they plan to buy for the baby, or all the ways they have heard of labour starting. In time, you can try more adventurous topics. Of course, what *you* think is a straightforward topic can and does bring all kinds of responses, so be prepared to be surprised!

Judging the level of group comfort and intimacy takes practice. One of the best clues is to pay attention to your own feelings – are you starting to relax with them, or is it still hard work to get them going? Pay attention to the group. Observe their body language – tense and anxious, or settled and at ease? How are they dealing with silences – able to leave them for a bit, or still rushing in to fill any spaces you leave? Are they beginning to listen to each other with interest, turning to look when someone speaks and following the next person's response? Have they started to volunteer information, including their feelings and beliefs? How have the rest reacted? Changes in their behaviour mirrors changes in how they are feeling within the group.

The role of the leader

Many groups discuss well without a leader. You still need to keep an eye on the general atmosphere, assessing the level of energy in the room and watching for signs of anxiety or boredom. If there are several small groups working at the same time, would they benefit from a discreet visit to check that everyone feels safe and at ease, or are they doing very well on their own? Listen for drops in the noise level that might signal the time to draw things to a close.

At other times you will want take part in discussions as a member of the group, albeit one with the special role as the leader. If the group seems unwilling to let you stop taking the lead, help them by reflecting back their questions – 'That's interesting ... anyone have some thoughts on that?'.

Acknowledge requests for information and postpone them for later. Instead of correcting misinformation yourself, you could invite others to offer their thoughts or experiences and continue to ask open questions.

Sometimes the behaviour of one or more group members prevents good discussion. You will find suggestions on how to handle this in Chapter 19.

Managing strong feelings

Sometimes a discussion allows parents to acknowledge or express deep feelings and worries. People may cry, become angry, or express great joy during the course of a discussion, allowing others to see how they really feel. The important thing to remember is that discussions do not *cause* these feelings; they may just provide a rare opportunity for them to be expressed (Figure 7.1).

Strong feelings and negative thoughts are worth airing because they tend to fester if left unspoken or buried at the back of people's minds. By allowing people to express their feelings, and maybe to cry, you are offering them a chance to let off steam, release their emotions and begin to hold the issue up to the light so that they can look at it with some perspective.

There are several things you can do to help individual members and the group as a whole to feel safe and supported, both during the expression of powerful feelings and afterwards as the group moves on:

- Stay looking calm.
- Acknowledge what is happening calmly and sympathetically.
- If it is appropriate, move closer to the person who is expressing strong feelings, to offer support rather than to stop him or her.

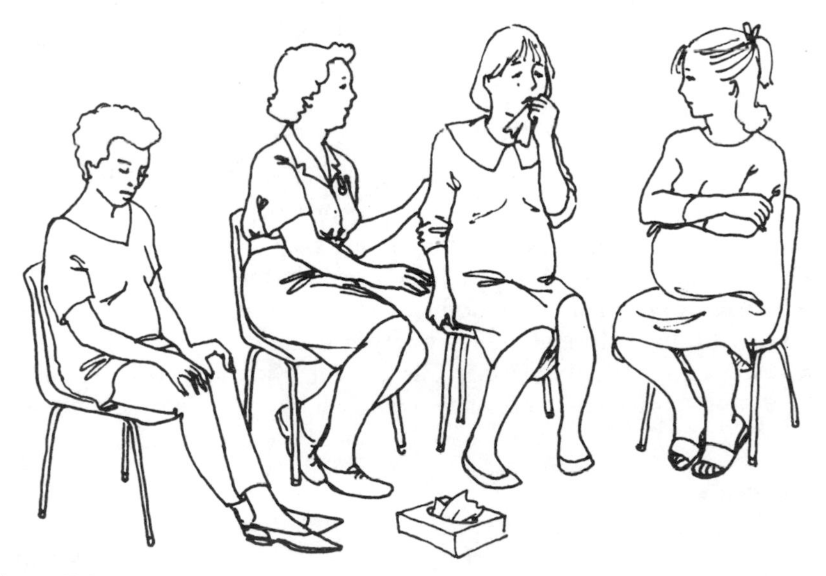

Figure 7.1

- Remember, tears can be infectious; if one person starts to cry, others might well join in.
- Avoid the temptation to reassure. If their fears are totally unfounded, you can put them into perspective later.
- Allow time, balancing the needs of the individual with those of the group.
- If someone leaves the room in distress, put people in small groups to talk about how they feel. This leaves you free to go out and offer support.
- If necessary, offer the individual time after the class to talk further.
- Afterwards, acknowledge what has happened. If the discussion has been hard for an individual or a group, it helps to say so briefly and with empathy. Then do something positive and active that involves everyone, so that the atmosphere lightened (for example, see the 'Advert for parents of a newborn baby' in Chapter 9).

Ending discussion

It is usually better to stop too soon rather than too late. Aim to end discussions before they peter out into uncomfortable silences. However, there may be occasions when the discussion takes too much time or goes way off the point, and you may then have to stop people in full flow. One way of doing this is to say, politely but firmly, 'I'm going to stop you there because we really need to move on to some of the other things you asked about'.

Initiating and maintaining discussion is like an adventure. You cannot predict what will happen. Like adventures, discussions can carry risks, but the benefits, giving people time to share their feelings and develop their thoughts and ideas, are well worth the effort.

Key points

- Discussions offer benefits that cannot be achieved in any other ways.
- Discussion is a good way of including everyone, valuing parents' views and experiences, and keeping people alert.
- The optimum size of group depends on what you want to achieve. If the topic is personal and emotive, form small groups; if you want to pool ideas and information, form larger groups.
- It is important to give participants a clear brief, ask good open questions, and tell people in advance what will happen after the discussion.

References

Bligh, D. (1998). *What's the Use of Lectures?*, 3rd edn, pp. 53, 67–8. Intellect.

Chapter 8

Teaching aids

This chapter discusses aids that not only provide a visual image, but also involve other senses such as sound and touch.

Well-chosen teaching aids can be powerful. They can enhance people's understanding and convey complex information quickly and simply. However, *describing* teaching aids simply and succinctly is not easy – proof that a picture is worth a thousand words. In this chapter we have done our best to convey in words what we would much prefer to show you. We hope that, with a bit of practice and with colleagues as your guinea pigs, you will be able to translate what we describe into vivid and memorable teaching techniques.

There is a huge variety of teaching aids, so you need to be selective. We suggest that you consider the following points.

- Keep them simple. Effective teaching aids do not have to be complicated or expensive.
- Use a few well-chosen aids, and remember that you are by far the most effective and reliable teaching aid of all.
- Whenever possible, use everyday things. By starting with something familiar and comparing it with something new, you increase understanding. You also reduce the chance that parents will concentrate on the aid itself rather than on the information you want to convey.
- Keep everything you use neat and clean. Grubby, tatty or incomplete aids are off-putting and worse than no aids at all. If you use written cards, make sure the writing is clear and legible; if you use pictures, make sure they are up to date and kept clean and neat. You may find it useful to mount written information and pictures on cards and cover them with transparent plastic. Shared equipment presents a particular challenge. Most parent education cupboards contain a tangle of teaching aids in various stages of disrepair. It is unwise to rely on finding what you want in a usable state. Plan ahead, sort out and clean up what you want to use – or, even better, create and bring in your own personal set of teaching aids.

- Parents need to be able to identify with the dolls, pictures and posters you use, so make sure that your teaching aids reflect the cultures and ethnicities of the people in your class.

Using your own body

Using your body expressively and imaginatively will help parents grasp and remember the concepts you introduce. You can do this in several ways.

Illustrating on yourself

Link what you are describing to your own body. For example.

- Stand sideways and hold life-size charts up against you (see Figure 8.1).
- Indicate the length and location of a Caesarean scar with a neat, small gesture on your own body.
- Show where your diaphragm, coccyx, pubic symphysis and pelvic brim are, before encouraging parents to find theirs.
- Hold the doll up against your own body to show lie and engagement.

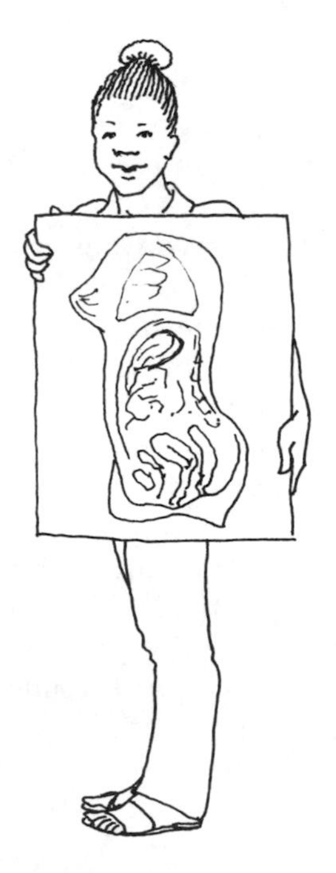

Figure 8.1

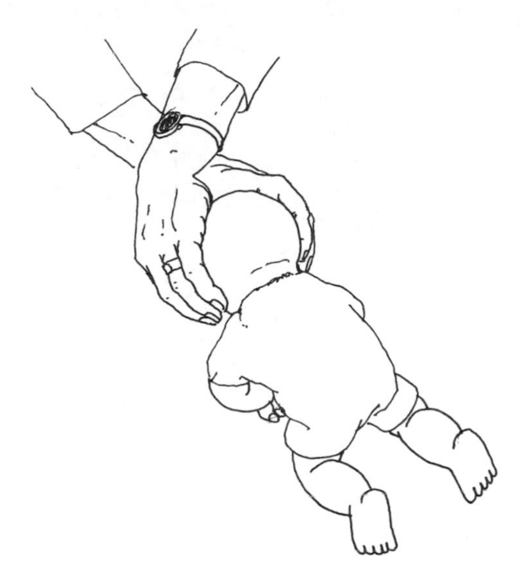

Figure 8.2

Demonstrating an action

Making your actions as realistic as possible helps people to remember. Thus, when you are showing how to get back in bed after a Caesarean section, demonstrate the effort and discomfort (and don't forget to breathe out and drop your shoulders when it 'hurts').

Many common procedures are easily adapted to mime.

- Your cupped hands can become two forceps blades. Place a doll in front of you, feet facing away, then slide your cupped right hand along the left side of the doll's head, copying the usual actions of whoever is applying the forceps. Do the same with your left hand along the right side of the doll's face (note that your wrists are now crossed), and 'lock' your elbows. You can demonstrate the position of the forceps on the baby's head by putting your hands on your own head (see Figures 8.2, 8.3).
- Instead of *talking* about posture in pregnancy, try tying a doll onto your body using a stretchy shawl. Adopt the arched back and wide-based walk of a heavily pregnant woman. Ask the group, 'what is supporting the baby?', and show how the stretch of the shawl from your back and down either side of the baby mimics the ligaments that often ache in pregnancy. Then demonstrate correct posture and pelvic rocking. To tie the doll in place, fold the shawl into a triangle and place it on your lap with the point facing away from you. A knitted or crocheted shawl about one metre square works best. Put the doll, head towards your body, on the shawl. Bring the point of the shawl up towards your chest so that the doll lies head down against your body and is completely covered by the shawl. Then tie the long ends of the shawl around your

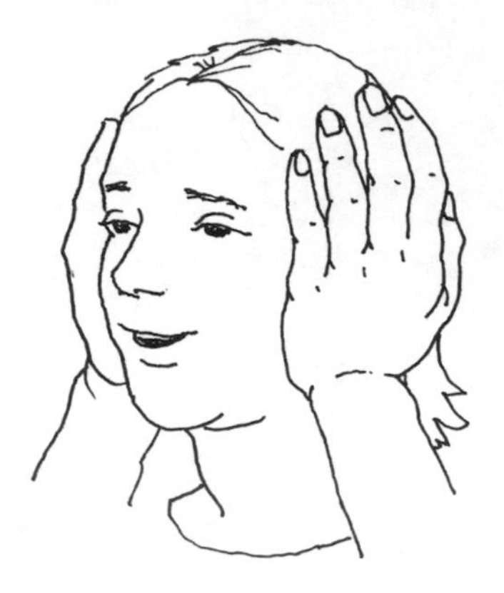

Figure 8.3

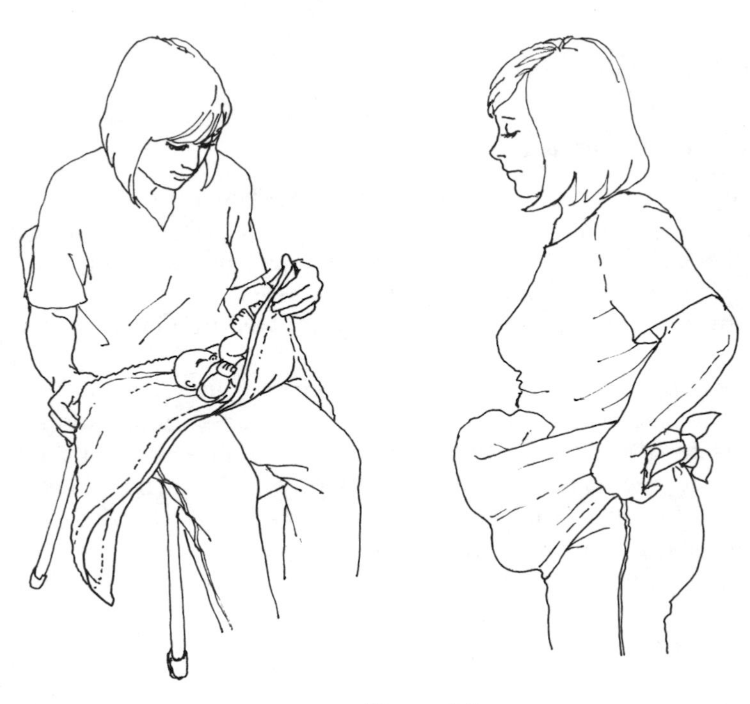

Figure 8.4

Figure 8.5

body, with the knot as nearly as possible over your sacro-iliac joints, and tuck the pointed end over the doll's bottom. Before you stand up, make sure the baby is well tucked in so that you do not leave an indelible memory of a precipitate birth (see Figures 8.4 and 8.5).

- Push your thumb between the second and third fingers of your clenched fist, and you have a satisfactory 'nipple' (see Figure 8.6).
- Drawing two hands gradually back over your bowed head until they

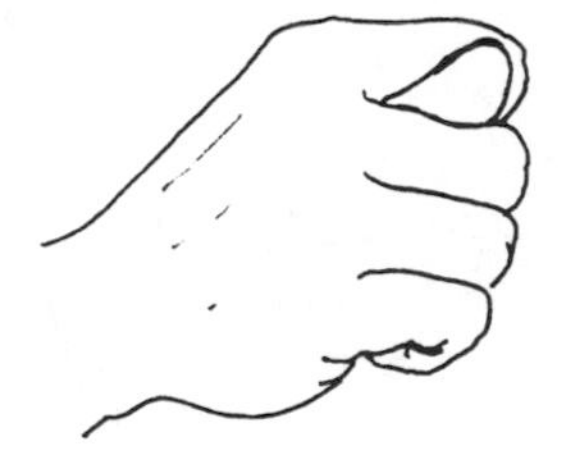

Figure 8.6

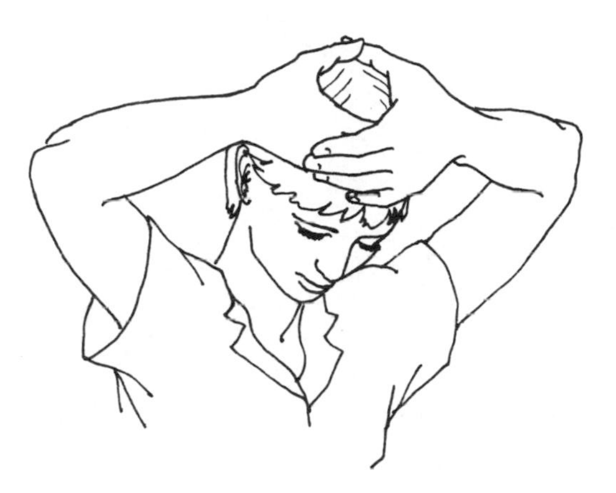

Figure 8.7

rest around your ears will translate dilatation from an abstract notion to something real and tangible (see Figure 8.7).

- Stretch your thumb and first finger widely apart. The arch of skin between them can be used to simulate the perineum. Point thumb and fingers upward, and use the fist of your other hand as the baby's head. You can also draw a circle below the arch of skin to represent the anus, and perhaps add a J-shaped line to show the position and shape of an episiotomy (see Figure 8.8).

Acting

Once parents understand the mechanics of a contraction, you can paint a more realistic picture by adding the sounds of labour. Try a groan, whimper slightly, catch your breath with a sharp pain, and then breathe out, drop your shoulders and let the contraction happen. Add the look of labour – turn your attention away from the room, drop your head, rock from side to side and so on.

You can do the same with the second stage, demonstrating the last three or four contractions that lead up to the baby's birth. Start by wrapping the doll in a shawl, tucking it under your arm, and placing your hands over

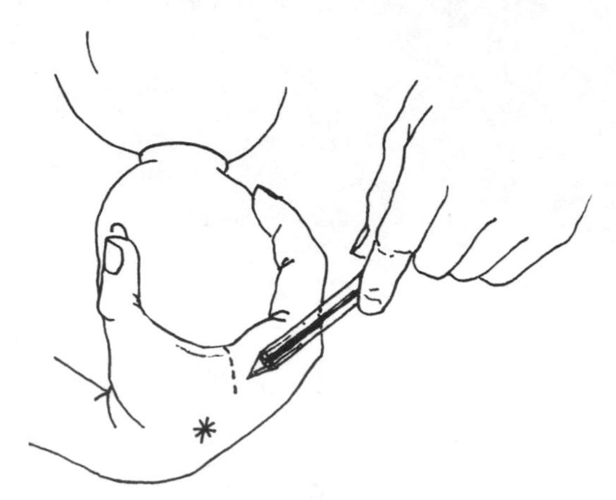

Figure 8.8

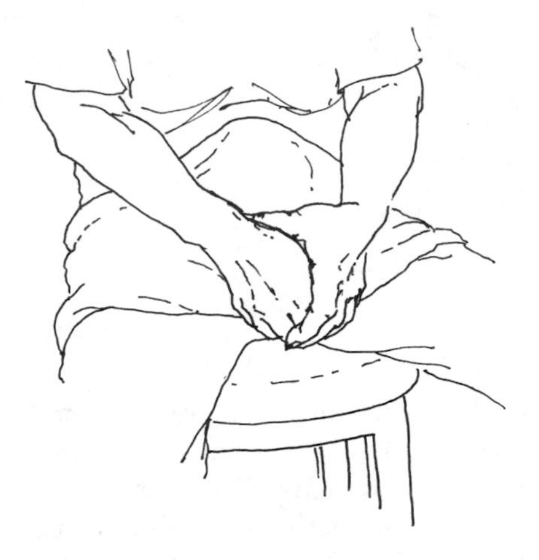

Figure 8.9

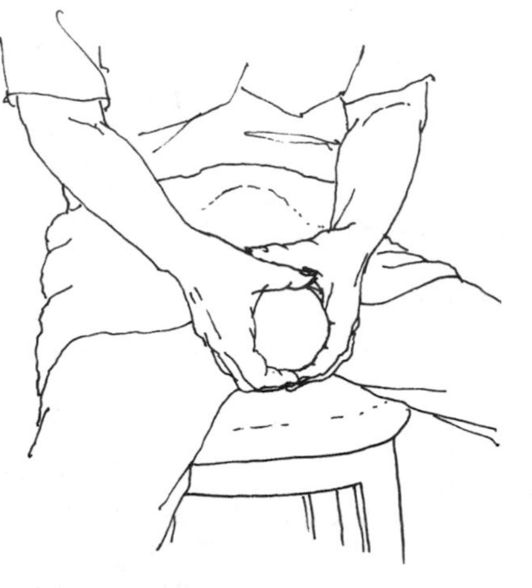

Figure 8.10

the head to form the vulva. Then simulate the gradual gape of the vulva and the emergence and retreat of the baby's head by moving your hands over the doll's head. Rest between contractions and show how, with each contraction, more and more of the head appears. Demonstrate crowning, panting as the baby's head emerges. Then show how the baby turns and, with one more push for the shoulders, slithers out. You can then cuddle the baby and ask them how they plan to welcome their own.

As you become confident you can add the sounds and facial expressions of a woman pushing, and, instead of holding the doll under your arm, place it on your tummy, covered with a shawl so that the head emerges from between your legs (see Figures 8.9 and 8.10).

We would encourage you to develop your acting ability; however, you will need to practise and have a sense of humour about your early efforts! Save the sounds of pain and panic until you feel more confident, the group members feel comfortable with each other, and you have a sense of what will and will not work. You will probably discover, as we have, that parents identify so closely with what you are doing that they almost believe they are witnessing the real thing and get a glimpse of how they might feel and react. You can tailor your demonstration to the group's reactions, adjusting your speed or stopping to answer questions. You can also add a joke or two if the atmosphere becomes a bit too intense – 'I'm progressing well ... how are you doing?' ... ' I have very short second stages – I'm sure you won't mind!'.

Involving the whole class

Here are two examples of how parents can be invited to be their own teaching aids.

Finding out about the pelvis

A plastic pelvis is commonly used in classes. However, it has several disadvantages. Parents often spend time wondering whose it once was, and as soon as you put it down it is at the 'wrong' angle, giving an inaccurate impression of the passage the baby takes. An alternative is to help everyone to discover their own pelvis and, in the process, recap or learn some technical words and understand the structure of the pelvis from a subjective rather than an objective standpoint. You can demonstrate the passage that the baby takes during labour, and go on to discuss hormone changes, moulding, positions for labour, and pelvic floor exercises.

Demonstrate on yourself as you talk so that they can see as well as hear what to do, and so that you are the focus of attention. Keep it light and chatty. It helps to acknowledge that this is a strange thing to do, and to tell them that previous classes have found it useful. Invite everyone to participate. Include men if they are present; however, it is worth saying that the female pelvis is specially adapted to give birth, and that the internal space is bigger than theirs.

Have the parents sitting comfortably on their chairs and ask them to feel their own hip bones – iliac crests. Next, use your own hands to demonstrate that what they are feeling is the equivalent of your fingertips (see Figure 8.11). You could point out that the shape and angle of this part of the pelvis (represented by your hands and fingers) is not really important, but the space between your wrists and down towards your elbows is, because this is the passage that the baby takes. Women who look narrow hipped can have just as much space as those who appear to have broad hips.

Ask them to feel the bone at the base of their tummy/below the bump – the pubic bone. It helps to reduce tension if you suggest they don't press

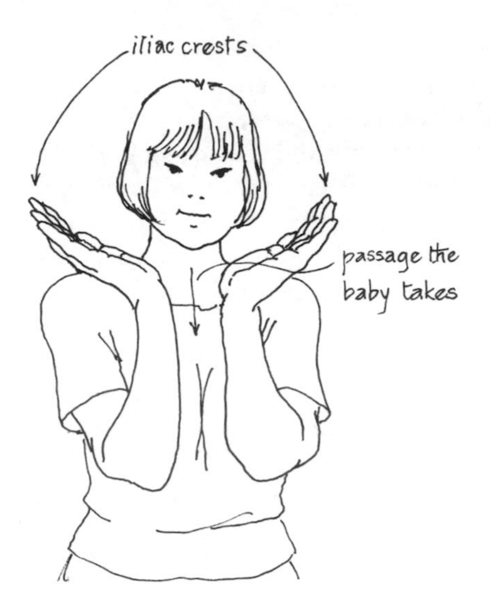

Figure 8.11

too hard in case their bladder is full! You could ask if any of the women find this spot sore or tender, and explain why this happens. You can point out that this bone forms the front of the pelvis, and that the baby's head will pass behind it.

Next ask them to slide their other hand down their back towards their tailbone and continue until they are sitting on their hand with their fingers pointing towards the front of their chair. Explain that what they are feeling is the back of the pelvis, and the baby travels in front of it. You could invite them to notice how the hand they are sitting on is curved. You can use your own hand to demonstrate the curve at the back of the pelvis, and a fist to show how the baby's head follows the curve during birth (see Figure 8.12).

Next you could ask them to stand, *but make sure you stand in the middle first* so that you are the centre of attention. Ask them to place one hand on their pubic bone and the other on their tailbone, just as they did before, and notice the space between them. Then invite them to bend their knees slightly and gently lean forward from the hips, and notice what happens to the space between their hands. Most people will discover for themselves that changing position increases the space. You could build on this by discussing the implications for labour and how certain positions can help – but ask them to sit down before you start a discussion!

You can follow this by suggesting that they sit on their hands, palms upwards, and see if they can feel their 'sitting' or ' butt' bones (see Figure 8.13). Parents do not have to stand to do this; they can remain seated and simply slide their hands under their bottom. Point out that their 'sitting bones' form the sides of the pelvis, and that the baby passes between them. Ask the women if they think this space feels small or big. If they

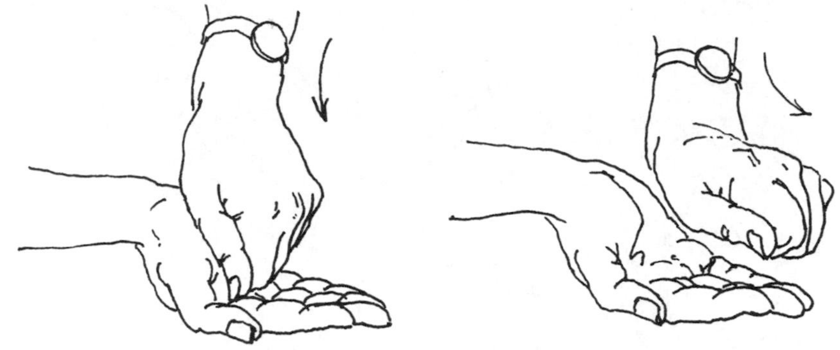

Figure 8.12

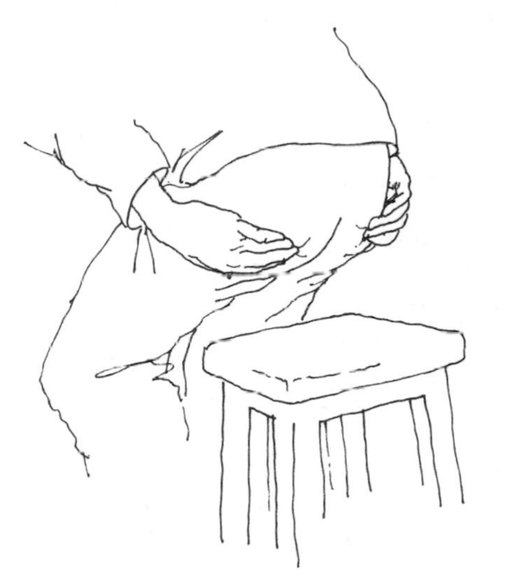

Figure 8.13

say small, you can remind them about the potential for the pelvis to expand and discuss how the baby's head moulds and adapts. You could follow this with pelvic floor exercises, since, whether they think the space is small or large, they now know that there is a space and that something must be supporting everything.

The first stage

You can model and involve everyone in a demonstration of the whole of the first stage. Invite everyone, men and women, to stand in a circle and join in. You could encourage the men by explaining that it helps the women; they cannot see their own hands under their bumps so they need to see what other people are doing (see Figure 8.14).

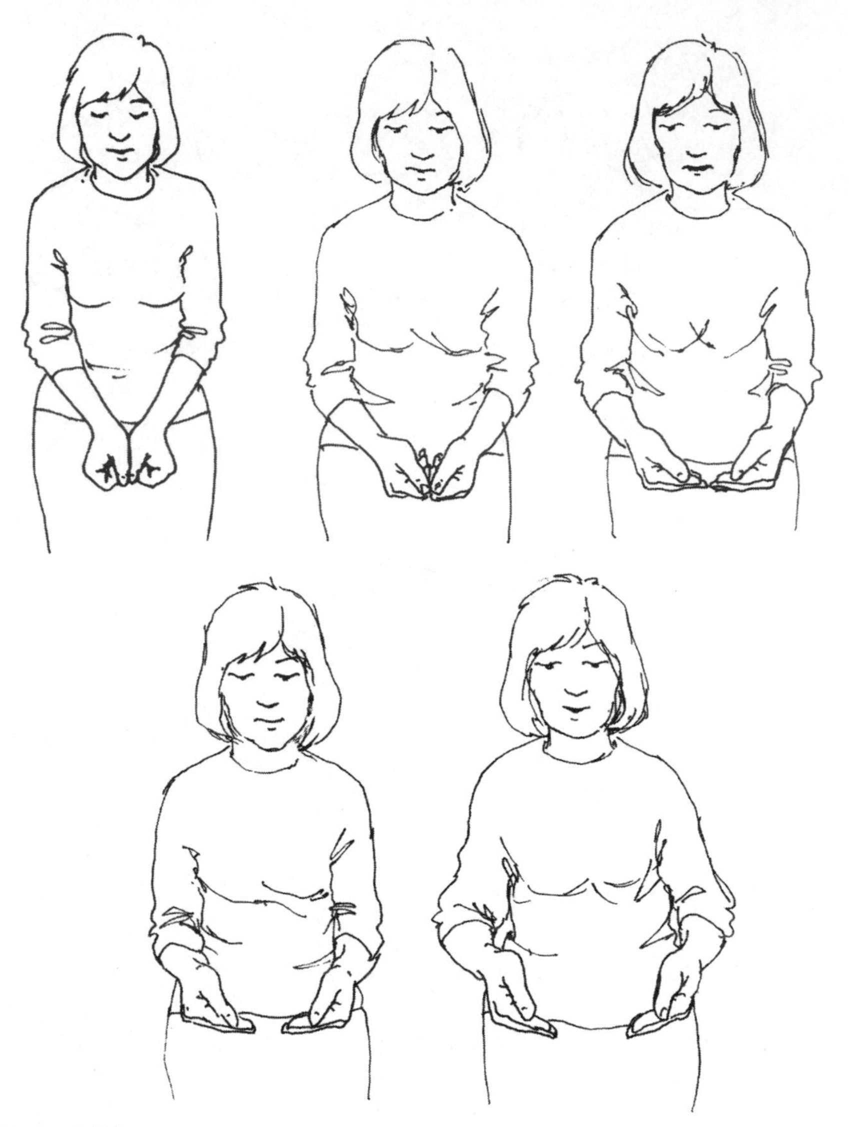

Figure 8.14

Talk them through a 'first stage', demonstrating as you go so that they can see as well as hear what you want them to do. Here is a sample script for you to use as a basis for telling your own story of the first stage.

Make fists with your hands – put them firmly together, with your thumbs parallel, and place them over the bottom of your belly (over your pubic bone). Your hands are like the cervix or neck of the uterus or womb. There is a plug of mucus down the centre, like a stopper in the bottle. Your arms are forming the sides of the uterus or womb in which your baby lies protected, safe and warm.

Towards the end of pregnancy the cervix starts to soften or ripen, thin and shorten (effacement). There is more room for the baby to sink down, become engaged. Drop your wrists slightly apart ... now flatten your hands a little so that just your knuckles are together, and uncurl your fingers so that just the tips are touching. The cervix is now completely thinned or effaced. This process can take several days, and at some point the plug of mucus – the show – may become detached.

Now pull your fingertips slightly apart, just enough so that a pencil tip would fit between them. The cervix is starting to open or dilate. Now a little bit more, so that there would be room for the pencil itself to fit in between, and now wide enough for a felt-tip pen. This process can take several hours or a day or so, and is called the latent phase. The woman may be getting backache and/or tummy tightening, and can feel restless and uncomfortable.

Once the cervix is about one and a half inches or four centimetres dilated, the woman is said to be in active labour. Now move your fingertips about two inches or five centimetres apart. This is about half way. Several more hours, say four or five, will have passed, and contractions have usually settled down into a regular pattern, getting longer, stronger and closer together as time passes.

Contractions are now getting really strong, lasting about 45 seconds and coming every five minutes, increasing to around 55 seconds every three minutes. Move your hands a little further apart, about three inches or seven centimetres. After about 12–14 hours, there are only three more centimetres to go!

Another hour or so, and the cervix is about three and a half inches or nine centimetres dilated. Some women may start to feel pressure on their back passage as the baby's head moves down, getting ready to be born. Now move your fingertips about 4 inches or 10 centimetres apart. The cervix is now fully dilated, wide enough for the baby's head to fit through, and the second stage can start.

As you develop this activity you may want to add other topics – for example, when to go into hospital or call the midwife, and what will happen on admission. Once everyone has completed effacement, you can highlight the change by putting your hands back as fists and comparing them to someone standing next to you. You can demonstrate how the baby's head descends by placing your fist above the hands of the woman standing next to you. At the same time, with the person's permission, you can demonstrate how two fingers are used to assess the dilatation during internal examinations. Make sure, however, that you do not demonstrate on a man!

Modelling sensations

As well as sights, you can model sensations. Ask everyone to put their fingers in both corners of their mouth and pull gently sideways. Feel the stretch? Then a bit harder ... and a bit harder? Usually, people describe their lips as hot and tingly; some mention pain and fear; most say their lips feel numb and cold when they let go. The parallels with crowning are obvious and enlightening.

Your teaching doll

After your own body, a teaching doll is the most important visual aid you can have. It may take some effort to find the ideal doll, but it will be time well spent. A good doll must be attractive and look as much like a real baby as possible. *Obstetric dolls should never be used with parents*. There are several 'teaching dolls' on the market; however, you may find a cheaper and more attractive doll in your local toyshop.

Most toy dolls are sold fully clothed and securely packaged. Insist on having them unpacked and undressed before you make your choice. We have seen dolls that look sweet when dressed, but decidedly unnatural when naked. Choose a doll with a nice face and a well-shaped body that is soft and flexible to the elbows and knees. Your doll does not need to be exactly the same size as a newborn baby. However, if you intend to put your doll through a pelvis, take a pelvis with you and make sure the doll fits through without a struggle! (We have found shop assistants helpful but quizzical when we have done this.) Ideally, your doll should also feel right when you cuddle it. If the body is very firm, try removing a little stuffing to get that floppy feel. Choose dolls that parents can identify with. In a multi-ethnic area, have a black doll as well as a white one.

Always treat your doll like a real baby. Wrap it in a shawl, keep it tucked up in a padded box or basket, and wash it and its blankets regularly to keep it pristine. When you handle your doll, talk to it and apologize for any awkward manoeuvres. Make sure you cradle the head when you wrap and unwrap it, and put it gently 'back to sleep' when you are finished. In this way you are not only helping parents to visualize their own baby, you are also teaching parenting skills. This may be the first time that some parents have seen a 'baby' held lovingly, in a variety of positions, comforted, winded. For most observers, within seconds your teaching doll *is* a baby. Their gasp of horror should you forget and handle the doll roughly or fling it into its box will be proof of their identification.

Make your own aids

Placenta and cord

If you want a placenta and cord, the cheapest option is to make your own. Cover a dinner plate-sized piece of two-and-a-half centimetre thick sponge rubber with dark red material such as towelling (the knobblier the better). Buy three one-metre lengths of thick cord from a haberdashery department (dressing gown cord or the kind used to tie back heavy curtains), one scarlet, the other two darker red or purplish to mimic veins and arteries. Twist or plait the lengths together and fix them by tacking with needle and thread. Unravel one end of the plaited cord and fan the strands out across the surface of your cloth 'placenta' and stitch in place. Encase the cord with fabric from a pair of sheer pale-grey tights. Sew one half of a press stud onto the free end of the twisted cord and the other half of the press stud onto the doll's tummy to make a 'navel'. Now you can attach and detach the cord.

A perineum

You can make a model of a perineum from a plastic kitchen bowl. Cut a hole in the bottom large enough to fit your doll's head easily, and then cut a circle of thin foam rubber larger than the hole and lay it in the bottom of the bowl. It will fit better if you glue and shape the foam so it is bowl-shaped too. Cut a cross-shaped opening in the foam rubber big enough to accommodate the doll's head without tearing. When using the contraption, put it between your knees at about the angle of a woman's pelvis.

By pushing against the bottom of the bowl with your doll's head, you can mimic a bulging perineum and crowning head of the end of the second stage. Your actions and noises can make this in some ways more realistic. Some class leaders put the doll inside a plastic bag (explaining to the group that this is just the purpose of the demonstration), as the resulting shiny wet appearance echoes the membranes.

Everyday items

There are endless everyday things that can illustrate and enhance the information you give. Here are some examples:

- *'Embryos'*. You can show the size and growth of the 'baby' in the early weeks of pregnancy by using a grain of pudding rice (the size at three weeks' gestation), a black-eyed bean (the size at four weeks'), a kidney bean (the size at six weeks'), a broad bean (the size at eight weeks') and a dried fig (the size at twelve weeks' gestation). Pass these tiny 'babies' around, cradling them gently. Invite discussion on what it felt like to hold such a tiny being, and talk about the rapid rate of growth and what the babies could do at those different stages of growth.

- *Balloons*. Blow them up full, slap on a lick-and-stick parcel label with 'placenta' written on it, let half the air out and watch the label buckle and detach. This is the ideal beginning to a discussion about the third stage.
- *Freezer bag clips*. These make excellent re-useable cord clamps.
- *Fruit*. A bunch of grapes illustrates the anatomy of the breast. Bananas demonstrate the curve through which the baby travels during the second stage, and give women a picture of the direction in which the baby travels. A pear, cut longitudinally, looks like a just-pregnant uterus.
- *A drive belt from an upright vacuum cleaner*. This is useful to demonstrate a fully dilated cervix, because most are 10 centimetres across and they are stretchy.
- *An egg cup*. An egg cup that holds around 30 cubic centimetres of fluid provides an indication of the capacity of a newborn infant's stomach (Davies and Davies, 1962). Combined with the knowledge that the baby doubles his or her birth weight by six months, this image helps to explain the need for frequent feeds.
- *A small natural sponge*. This can be cut to size so that it absorbs about 30 cubic centimetres of water, and can be squeezed out to show how much a newborn baby's stomach can hold.
- *A ruler*. This helps parents to internalize the distance at which a newborn baby can focus, and helps to provide a visual image of building a relationship with a new baby. Hold the doll as if you are breastfeeding, and use the ruler to show that the distance between the baby's face and yours is about 9–12 inches (22–30 centimetres). Using the doll and ruler, show how, if parents hold an alert newborn baby in front of them, the baby can focus on their face (see Figure 8.15).
- *A polo neck sweater*. This provides an effective way of demonstrating how the position of the baby affects the progress of labour, and works particularly well because it draws on people's existing knowledge and experience. Choose a polo neck suitable for an 18-month-old baby – any stretchy fabric will do. Demonstrate how the baby lies head down inside the sweater or 'uterus' and how the polo neck forms the cervix (for anatomical accuracy, the arms are like the Fallopian tubes). Next ask the class to think about putting on a polo neck sweater. Most will say that they usually drop their chins a little in order to pull the sweater over the dome-shaped part of their heads. You can point out that this helps the polo neck to stretch easily and evenly, and that it is much more of an effort to pull it on over the top or front of the head. Next, take the doll out of the sweater so that you can show against your own body how a baby in an anterior position is able to curl up so that the dome-shaped part of the head is in contact with the cervix. Then show

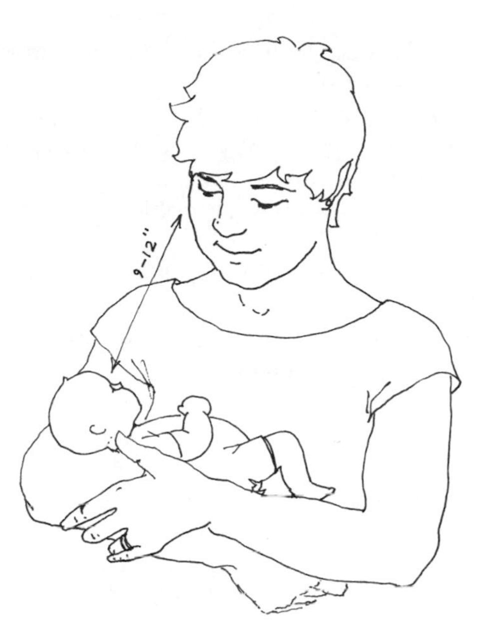

Figure 8.15

how a baby in a posterior position cannot curl up, so the cervix is likely to take longer to dilate.

The real thing

Collect and pass around things that parents might encounter or use during labour and birth. A range of items such as an amnihook, a CTG trace, an Entonox mouthpiece, forceps and cord clamps are commonly brought into classes and handed round for people to touch and examine. When making your choice, think carefully about your reasons for including each item. Bear in mind that, unless parents ask for clinical details, you are preparing them for subjective experiences and not clinical technicalities. Will the item enlighten and help them to cope with the experience, or will it only serve to raise anxiety? For example, do parents need to know about the different types of forceps? Will seeing a trochar and cannula for an epidural increase the aversion that many women have to the thought of having anything inserted into their back. Might they be reassured by seeing and handling an epidural catheter and knowing that they will not spend hours with a needle in their back?

You can also use real sounds – tapes of a baby crying and crying, or a grizzly baby; an actual birth; the first greeting between mother, father and baby; womb sounds; a noisy sucking baby and so on. These can be used on their own, or added to relaxation and visualization exercises as appropriate.

Photographs of techniques and equipment are almost as good as the real thing. So, too, is a series of photographs that tell a story – e.g. the same baby photographed six or seven times during a feed, or a series of photographs demonstrating a baby's 'milestones'. The photographs should be large, perfectly in focus, clear and up to date. If you have no good ones, contact your nearest photographic club or sixth form college to find a photographer willing to take a series as a project.

If you want to use a photograph more than once, mount it and cover it with transparent plastic. Alternatively, you can use drawings. Parents will welcome the chance to handle, inspect and pass these around themselves. This helps them to establish ownership of the information – a process made more difficult if the teacher holds onto everything.

Charts and diagrams

There is a range of charts and diagrams on the market, or you can devise your own. Here are some points to bear in mind when choosing and using charts and diagrams:

- If you have a set of diagrams or charts, look at them critically and use only those that really illustrate the points you want to cover.
- Most people are not familiar with cross-sections of anatomy. Choose uncluttered pictures that show clearly what you want to explain.
- Make sure that the charts and details you point out are clearly visible to everyone in the room.
- Help people to orientate themselves by identifying landmarks that you have already talked about – 'here is the pubic bone and here's the tailbone'.
- Where possible, use life-size diagrams and hold them against your body in the correct position so they can see where the part fits into the whole.
- If charts that demonstrate a process rather than a single event (for example, changes during pregnancy or labour) are ring-bound, you can only show one at a time. If you mount them separately, you can line them up and compare them. This allows people to see the progressive changes that take place.
- When using charts to show the progress of the baby during labour, hold them upright rather than horizontally. This demonstrates the benefits of being upright and mobile during labour.

Posters

Attractive posters can brighten a room and convey useful images and messages. To be effective, posters need to:

- be changed regularly. It is easy to tell if a particular poster has been there for ages. As soon as the viewer realizes this, the message loses impact
- reflect the lifestyles, cultures and ethnicities of the people they are aimed at. White middle-class images are easy to find, but can alienate people who do not identify with them
- offer carrots, not sticks. Effective posters meet parents' needs and help them to feel positive and good about themselves
- be carefully selected so that people are not overwhelmed by them. We have worked in rooms plastered with posters, even finding several at eye level for the 'captive audience' in the toilet.

So stand back and take a critical look at your walls. If you came into the room for the first time, would it look friendly and attractive, or does it look too busy? Are the messages bossy, or do they require too much effort to take in? Are they alienating? We recently worked in a parent education room that had a display about the history of midwifery. This included a photo of a heavily pregnant woman lying supine whilst a midwife wielded a huge pair of fearsome looking calipers to measure the fundal height!

Some posters need no words at all. One parent education room we worked in had a collage of dozens and dozens of snapshots of newborn babies, each labelled with his or her name on a small card in the lower left corner – Alex, Isabelle, Deepak, Katy, Mercy. That poster's message was, 'babies are individual and different, and we love and value them all . . .'. The collage was unfinished, and a card in the empty lower right corner said, 'And we are waiting for yours'. You could also have collage of pictures and photographs of fathers holding, bathing and changing their babies. This says, 'fathers are important too, and have a lot to contribute and a lot to gain by sharing the care of their babies'.

Some posters need words. The simpler and more inviting the written message, the more likely it will be 'heard' and understood. Never use three words when one will do. Use an image instead of a word if you can. Search for memorable phrases. Finally, value white space, because it allows the eye to 'think'.

Videos

Videos have become an integral part of many antenatal courses, and many leaders feel they ought to show at least one. If you use or plan to use a video in your class, watch and listen to it critically.

- Does it include the information and ideas that you want to convey?
- Does it include messages or images that are outdated or unhelpful? Remember that however careful your verbal disclaimers are, you cannot erase an inaccurate or alarming visual image.

- Does the video convey the parents' perspective, or give the professional's view of events? A video that focuses on a larger-than-life bulging perineum can be upsetting. The mother will certainly not have this view of her own labour, and her partner is unlikely to either.
- Would watching this video be time well spent? Is it short enough to trigger activities and discussion, or would it take up valuable time that could be spent in more productive ways?

Although showing videos can have advantages, there are several drawbacks.

- Videos turn your group into an audience.
- It is hard to judge reactions when people sit in the dark facing a screen, and you cannot stop in the middle to respond to their concerns and anxieties.
- You are reliant on having the right equipment in working order. There is nothing more frustrating and embarrassing for everyone than wasting time on a malfunctioning TV, video or remote control.
- Many parents have already seen videos or TV programmes on birth, and are keen for something else. They often show this by talking through the video. A group that reacts in this way is telling you that they recognize the unique opportunity that being in an antenatal class offers them, and they are reluctant to spend it as a passive audience.
- Some parents are alarmed and put off by birth videos.
- Some dread the prospect of watching a video, and may even avoid classes because they do not want to see 'anything gory'.

If you find a suitable video that will enhance what you offer and be time well spent, you will need to find a way of balancing the needs of those that want to see a video and those that don't. One way to meet differing needs and expectations is to offer a video session as an add-on extra, so that those who want to can opt in and those who decide not to come do not lose out on class time.

Key points

- Well-chosen teaching aids enhance understanding, and can convey complex information quickly and simply.
- The cheapest, most available, flexible and most effective teaching aid is you. It's well worth setting aside your inhibitions and taking the risk of showing parents, to the best of your ability, what labour or feeding or caring for a new baby is really like.
- A well-chosen doll is extremely useful. *Obstetric dolls should never be used with parents.*

- Keep teaching aids simple. Everyday familiar things can be more effective than complicated and costly equipment.
- It is important to keep teaching aids spotlessly clean and neat.

References

Davies, D. V. and Davies, F. (eds) (1962). *Gray's Anatomy, Descriptive and Applied*, 33rd edn. Longmans.

Chapter 9

Active learning

This chapter discusses how and why to include active learning techniques in antenatal classes, and offers some practical examples.

Why use active learning techniques?

Classes that include a variety of activities that encourage people to identify what they already know, try things out for themselves and reflect on what they have heard are unlikely to be boring. When people take an active part in the learning process, they are more likely to feel empowered and to remember and use what they have learned (Bligh, 1998). They can frame further questions, consolidate what they have learned, and think about how they might use it in practice. They can also have fun.

Planning

Clarifying your purpose

Before choosing or designing active learning techniques for your class, decide what you want to achieve.

- Do you want to find out what they already know? For examples, see 'Paperchase' and 'Compare and contrast' below.
- Do you want to combine hearing, seeing and doing? Activities can be a good alternative to lectures, and people often absorb more information when they discover things for themselves. For examples, see 'Finding out about the pelvis' and 'The first stage' in Chapter 8, and 'The 24-hour clock' below.
- Are you aiming to reinforce and consolidate information that you have given them? For examples, see 'Is she in labour?' and the 'Labour line' below.

- Do you want to encourage people to think about what they would do in different situations? For examples, see 'Is she in labour?' and 'Situation cards' below.
- Are you using the activity to change the pace and atmosphere in the class? Activities such as the 'Paperchase' and the 'Advert for parents' (see below) are excellent for increasing alertness, raising energy and introducing a lighter note.

Laying the foundations

A class that has remained an audience will be far less likely to respond positively to an invitation to participate than a class that has already become a group. To feel like a group, people need to know each other, be used to contributing their thoughts and ideas, and above all be confident that any contribution they make will be accepted and welcomed. If you want active participation, you need to set the scene right from the beginning of the first class (see Chapter 5).

Ensuring relevance

Your activities will only be effective if they are relevant to the people in your class. Check that they reflect the cultures and lifestyles of your participants. Are they relevant to different socio-economic or ethnic groups? Are they appropriate for teenagers, single or adoptive parents? If you teach couples, is the partner's perspective included?

Demonstrating respect

If you want people to participate and continue to do so, the experience must be useful, positive and enjoyable for them. Avoid putting people on the spot. Never ask anyone to do something that has a right or wrong answer. Accept every response you get, adjusting it if necessary (see 'Adjusting information' below). You can help people to feel valued by thanking them after they have participated in an activity.

Relinquishing control

Some activities involve groups working on their own. This means that the role of the leader has to change. Once you have set up the groups and shown them what to do, you are no longer centre stage. You can have a short break and stand back and observe. However, this also means relinquishing control. This worries some class leaders, possibly because they cannot predict what will happen or keep a check on what is going on in each group, and because they fear that people might reach the 'wrong' conclusions.

Keeping a tight rein on the class may feel safer, but it denies participants opportunities to reflect, discuss and reach their own conclusions – something that they will have to do in the end anyway. Encouraging parents to think and do things for themselves demonstrates respect and trust for them, and is realistic preparation for the responsibilities of parenthood.

This does not mean that you should abandon them completely. Be available, and repeat the brief if people are uncertain about what to do. You could join each group briefly, and answer questions or make suggestions if necessary.

Introducing active learning

The way you introduce activities is important. Calling them 'games' may be unwise, because some people find the idea of playing games childish while others may feel manipulated. Think of ways of inviting people to try something new that will stimulate their interest and sound inviting. For example, to introduce *'Is she in labour?'* (see below), you could say, 'We've talked about how labour starts, now let's look at it in a different way'. A positive and confident tone of voice is probably as important as the words you use.

Dividing the class

Activities should include everyone. Some can be used with the whole class together, while others need to be done in small groups. You need to work out the numbers in your class, and divide them into groups that are the appropriate size for the activity. If everyone in each group is involved throughout the activity, the groups can be larger – say six to eight people. If each person or couple has a turn while others observe, the group size should be smaller – say three to four – to avoid boredom and time wasting (for ways of dividing the class, see Chapter 4).

Explaining the task

Explaining what you want people to do can be surprisingly difficult. The task may be perfectly obvious to you, but then you have devised it or used it before. However, it is completely new to the people in your class. Work out, in advance, exactly what you want people to do and what you are going to say. If you give verbal instructions, make short, clear statements. You can back these up by writing them on cards, one for each group, or on a flip chart. Alternatively, start by demonstrating what you want people to do before you divide them up into small groups.

A troubleshooting guide

If an activity does not work or if people are not doing what you expect them to do, you need to check several things:

- *Is the ice melted?* Activities only work when the ice has been melted, when parents are sufficiently gelled and have participated from the very beginning of the course.
- *Check your timing*. Is it too soon for this particular activity? Do the parents need information before doing it? Does it link in with the topics you have been dealing with? Would it work better towards the end of the course, when they know each other better?
- *Review the size of the groups*. Are they appropriate for the activity?
- *Is the relevance clear?* People will be more willing to try something new if they can see that it will be useful.
- *Is literacy an issue?* People who have problems with literacy seldom say so. If you think this might be an issue for some of the parents in your group, try activities that do not require literacy.
- *Check your understanding of the activity*. Have you tried it out successfully before? If not, are you clear about how it works and what it can achieve? Does it need re-thinking?
- *Check your brief*. As a rule of thumb, if people have not understood what you want them to do, you have not got the brief right. When this happens, try saying something like, 'I'm sorry – I didn't explain that very well. What I meant to say was . . .'. By taking personal responsibility you reduce the chances of people feeling stupid, resentful or 'put on the spot', and increase their willingness to start again.

However, if a group lands up doing something unexpected *but which is relevant and useful*, let it happen. Listen, watch and learn!

Developing activities

There is an infinite number of activities you can devise and adapt. It can be great fun and very rewarding to invent your own. Keep them simple, and think about the appearance of the materials (see Chapter 8).

Practice

Before you use an activity in class, try it out with a group of friends or colleagues and ask them to give you feedback. Did it achieve your aim? Did they enjoy it? What did they learn? Were your instructions clear? What improvements could you make?

Feedback

When you have tried an activity in class, take time to notice the reactions of the participants. You could also ask them what they got out of it. Then review and, if necessary, adapt what you are doing for next time so that it becomes more effective.

Examples of active learning

Below we describe a few tried and tested activities. You may have come across them or used them already, as they are now being used by health professionals throughout the UK. However, if they are new to you, we acknowledge that it is often difficult to work out how to lead an activity and to be sure that it will work when you have only read about it – proof that seeing and doing are usually more effective. They will probably make much more sense when you actually do them. Try them out with a group of friends or colleagues, following the instructions step by step. You will then have a better idea of their potential and how you might use or adapt them.

Is she in labour?

This activity offers people a chance to consolidate the information they have received, to think about how they will recognize the onset of labour and how they might feel and react, and what self-help techniques they could use. It also makes it clear that the onset of labour is seldom a single event but more of an unfolding process, and that labour is unpredictable.

Optimum group size. Three to four women or couples, so that each woman has a turn and everyone has an opportunity to watch two or three others have a turn.

Timing. After you have discussed the onset of labour. Allow about 10–15 minutes of class time. This includes your explanation, the activity, and question and answer time.

Materials. Identical sets of cards. Write one event or feeling that women might experience as part of the onset of labour on each card. For example, each set could consist of 12 cards, each card with one of the following words or phrases printed on it:

irregular contractions
diarrhoea
backache that comes and goes
strong contractions lasting 50 seconds
mild contractions every five minutes
mild contractions every 20 minutes
a show
sudden gush of waters
?wet knickers?
'ouch' with a contraction
feeling sick
want to push!
spurt of energy
feeling shaky

Notice that there are no 'right' or 'wrong' answers, that we have used everyday rather than technical language, and that the activity concentrates on the subjective experience rather than the clinical process.

Process. Give each group a set of cards. Each woman has a turn to use the whole set of cards. She shuffles them, holds the pack face down and turns the cards up, one a time, laying them out in a line coming directly towards her. (Having the line of cards literally coming at you creates an impression of a personal and urgent series of events, whereas cards laid out from left to right can be viewed much more dispassionately.)

Each time the woman turns up a card, her task is to decide what she might do. Would she rest or carry on as usual? Try a warm bath? Eat something? Have a back rub? Call her partner? Call the midwife? Or rush to hospital?

In a couples' class, her partner might also have views about what should be done, and this is a good opportunity for couples to understand each other's expectations and assumptions about how they will handle different situations. Others in the group might have suggestions, but ultimately the woman (and her partner) need to decide. Once she has decided she is in labour, she stops and hands the cards on to the next woman, who shuffles them before taking her turn.

Explaining the task. The best way of explaining the task is to demonstrate by laying out the cards one by one and deciding out loud with each one what you could do. Then divide the class into groups and let them try it out for themselves.

Some leaders have tried giving individual cards to different people and asking them what they would do if what was written on the card happened to them. This has limited value, as the onset of labour is usually an unfolding process rather than a single event. Parents will learn more if each woman uses the whole set of cards (see Figure 9.1).

Your role You can circulate around the groups, asking the woman who is currently laying out the cards how things are going and what she thinks she might do at each stage. If appropriate, you can add suggestions, reinforce information – ' if your waters go, please let us know' – and encourage her to think of self-help techniques.

If the 'want to push' card keeps coming up early on, you could suggest that they set it on one side. Alternatively, you could leave it in and, after the activity, tell the whole group three things about emergency childbirth and three things about labour when the baby is in a posterior position.

Paperchase

This enables you to find out what parents already know and to use this as a basis for what you tell them. It is an effective way of covering large and complex subjects, for example pain relief or intervention in labour. It is also good for raising energy levels in a quiet and sleepy group!

Optimum group size. You need three or four groups each of around five to eight people.

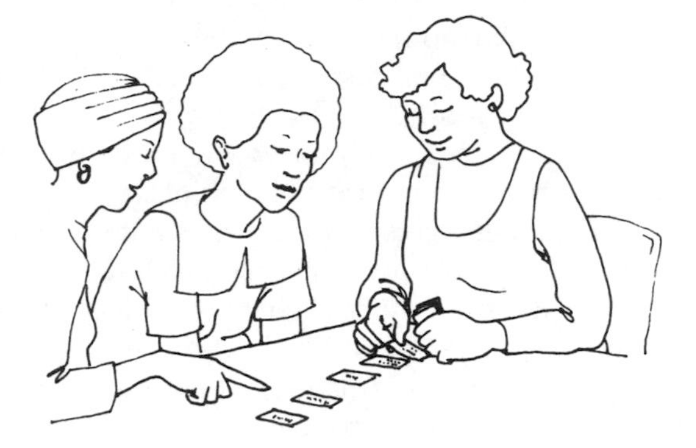

Figure 9.1

Timing. This works best if you use it as an introduction to the topic you wish to cover. The actual paperchase takes five to ten minutes. You also need about ten minutes per sheet for discussion and review.

Materials. You need a sheet of A1 paper and a felt-tip pen for each group. All the felt-tip pens should be the same colour in order to minimize comparisons and competition between the groups.

Process and your role. Divide your class into three or four groups, place a sheet of paper and a pen in the centre of each group, and ask them to choose a scribe. If you want to cover pain relief, you could allocate topics such as pethidine (or whichever opiate is used in your area), epidural and gas and oxygen. If you have four groups, you could add self-help for labour or TENS. If you choose intervention, you could allocate topics such as induction, forceps and Caesareans.

Give each group a topic and ask them to write it at the top of their sheet. Then ask them to write down everything they have *heard* about the topic on their sheet. Using the word *heard* rather than *know* reduces competition, removes the pressure to get it right, and allows parents to include things that they have been told but are not sure about. You may elicit half-truths and possibly old wives' tales, which gives you an opportunity to adjust the information so that their knowledge is factual and accurate (see 'Adjusting information' below).

If you want to raise energy as well as gather ideas, start by saying 'Ready, steady ... go!'. As soon as each group has at least two things written down, say loudly and firmly, 'Finish what you are writing and don't start another one!'. Then, as fast as you can, move the sheets (either clockwise or anti-clockwise) around the group! The more speed you use, the greater the energy rise. Ask them to look at their new topic, see what is on the sheet and add to it. Give them time to write three or four things and then move the sheets again, always in the same direction. Repeat the process until each group has written on every sheet and has its own sheet back again.

The speed of the moves is dictated by the rate at which people are working. You do not want to hand on an empty sheet, nor do you want one group to leave nothing for others to add. If one group is working faster than the others, take their sheet away first. This leaves other groups a few extra seconds.

You can now display each sheet, review what they have written down, and summarize by giving your three key points. People's concentration will be improved if you intersperse your reviews with something active. So after each summary, you could invite people to talk in small groups about how they feel about the topic in hand. What would they choose or do? You may want to encourage flexible attitudes. For example, 'How would you feel if there was no time to have an epidural?'; 'Suppose it looks like you will need forceps to help the baby turn to the right position?'.

Alternatively, do something active and relevant to the subject in hand. For example, if the subject is pain management you could practise positions for labour; if it is intervention you could suggest women try relaxing while lying down with a pillow across their chests to see what it might feel like to have a screen up during an epidural Caesarean.

Adjusting information. If you ask people to contribute, you must accept everything they say. If you do not, many people will be reluctant to speak out again. However, you also need to deal with misconceptions and ensure that parents have accurate and factual information. This can be achieved by:

- acknowledging what they say so that they feel they have been heard – 'It's good that your sister thought that pethidine was brilliant and that she was not bothered by any side effects'
- then adjusting it to a more realistic picture – 'Some people do find it helpful and others don't like it so much because ...'
- adding in further information – 'We know that it can affect the baby, who may ..., so we usually give the baby an injection of an antidote straight after birth'.

Compare and contrast

This is another way of inviting parents to identify what they already know, and can be used as a basis for discussion and information giving. Parents are invited to compare things that are already familiar with things such as labour or early parenting that are outside their experience. We have found that subjects such as Christmas, going on holiday or running a marathon work well, although interesting comparisons can be made with many other topics. Choose a topic that is likely to elicit issues that fit in with what you want to cover. For example, the marathon is a good introduction to learning skills for dealing with the stress and pain of labour; Christmas and going on holiday are good for practical, social and emotional issues (see samples below).

Timing. You can use this activity at any time. Allow around five minutes for eliciting and charting, and then follow on with discussion and review.

Materials. A flip-chart stand, paper and two different coloured felt-tip pens.

Optimum numbers. This can be done with groups of all sizes.

Process and your role. Divide your chart paper into two columns, heading one column 'LIKE' and the other 'UNLIKE'. Write your subject (Christmas, Marathon, Holiday) across the centre of the heading. Ask parents to say all the ways in which having a baby is like your chosen subject, and chart them in the LIKE column. Then ask them all the ways it in which having a baby is unlike your chosen subject, and chart these with a different coloured pen in the second column. Saying something like, 'You probably think this is a bit crazy, but have a go' can help to get them going.

As with any brainstorm, accept everything, though you may want to suggest that perhaps something applies to the other column. Once your list is completed, you can pick out and discuss some of the issues that the group has raised.

We have used this activity for many years, and are still sometimes surprised and delighted by what people come up with. Just to reassure you that it works, here are some samples. If your group is slow to contribute or misses something useful, you could add one or two things yourself. The results of this activity can spark off a great deal of discussion and reflection on a range of useful issues.

Christmas

Like	*Unlike*
exciting	can't drink
busy	physical pain
expensive	no fixed date
surprise package	no fixed length
relatives visit	can't always plan
not always happy	a baby is not just for Christmas
presents and cards	no refunds or exchanges
late nights	no rest afterwards
feels never-ending	life will never be the same again
glad when over	restricted food
magical	unpredictable
inevitable	no alcohol
thank you letters	can't unwrap early
exhausting	frightening
stressful	overspend continues
indigestion	no fixed date
not sure what you will get	? not an annual event
over in a day	
lots of shopping	

A marathon

Like	*Unlike*
long and hard	can't drop out
never again!	can't see the end
takes a long time	no fixed length
stamina	no fixed route (? via theatres)
very physical	no fixed date
painful	no practice runs
hot and sweaty	limited control
raised endorphins	new family member
thirsty	can have help (drugs, intervention)
cramp	no cheering crowds
exhaustion	private
increased breathing and heart rate	usually not an annual event
want to stop	not a spectator sport
achievement	unpredictable
might wear funny clothes	not a competition
stitch	a medal at the end!
all consuming	not much sleep afterwards
adrenaline rush	

Going on holiday

Like	*Unlike*
plan what to take	no fixed date
pack a suitcase	no fixed length
plan your route	no food
strange place	no alcohol
strange bed	no suntan
new people	painful
may not be like the brochures	hard work afterwards
send cards to family and friends	exhausting
expensive	sleepless nights
not how you expected it to be	cost continues
don't understand the language	no insurance
(travel) sickness	not relaxing
the end is worth the hassle of the journey	

Labour line

This activity offers parents an overview of labour, and a chance to consolidate what they have learnt and identify any further questions that they might have. It can also be used to convey a visual image of the fact that labour is long and unpredictable.

Optimum group size. Because everyone is actively involved throughout this activity, you can have groups of around six women or three couples.

Timing. After you have covered the whole of labour. A good time is towards the end of the course, perhaps at the start of the last class. Allow about 15 minutes if you want to include reflection and discussion.

Materials. Each group will need a pack of cards. Each card has written on it one thing that women might feel, experience or do during a normal labour. For example, you could have a card for each of the following:

Labour line – the mother

walking around
feeling fed up
hot and tingling perineum
backache
feeling hot
contractions 50 seconds long
thigh ache
so excited!
desperate for a cup of tea
feeling sick
have a bath
want to push
like listening to music
feeling sweaty
decide to go to hospital
HELP!
gas and oxygen
contractions 60 seconds long
don't want to be touched
severe back pain
contractions feel continuous
low back pain
can't go on
contractions every 10 minutes
scrambled eggs on toast
contractions stop
try leaning forward on a chair
feet feeling very cold
feeling frightened
ring up in-laws
contractions one minute long
hot water bottle to tummy
strong contractions
contractions 30 seconds long
sleepy between contractions
don't want to push
pushing
oh, lovely
shaky legs
had enough – want to go home
baby born
more pushing
feeling dizzy, try breathing slowly
period-type pains
diarrhoea
pressure on back passage
don't want to be left alone
panic
contractions every 3 minutes
exhausted
try all fours
walking around
what a relief

The large number of cards is deliberate as, once the task is finished, you are left with a strong visual message that labour is long – something that parents find hard to take in.

You can also include the labour partner's perspective. For example, you might have a set of cards with one of the following written on each card. Use a different coloured card for the partners so that their experience stands out when you review after the activity:

Labour line – the partner

exhausted	feeling tired	feeling nervous
feeling worried	lump in throat	sponge her face
make sandwiches	time to call the hospital?	offer a back rub
offer a massage	tea and a sandwich	get a breath of fresh air
excited	phone to say won't be in to work today	

Notice that there is no 'right' or 'wrong', that we have used everyday language, and that the activity deals with the subjective experience rather than the clinical process. We have not included obstetric interventions, because this would imply that these are routine and would also complicate the activity and risk people getting something 'wrong'.

The task. Each group places their cards on the floor in one long line, in the order that reflects their view of what might happen in labour. Everyone works together. Once the line is completed, ask the partners to share out the partner's cards and place them alongside the mother's line to indicate how they might feel and react to what is going on.

Explaining the task. It helps if you give instructions in stages so that parents can complete part of the task before hearing what to do next. Start by explaining that each group is going to use their set of cards to tell the story of a labour. Make sure that everyone knows where 'the labour' will start, and that all the groups are working in the same direction so that you land up with several parallel labour lines. It helps if you say something like, 'We'll have the onset of labour starting on this side of the room, working towards the birth on that side'.

You could then demonstrate by placing a small number of cards from one of the sets on the floor in a line. So, for example, if you have a card with 'walking around', place it near the start. 'severe backache' would go much further down the line, and 'baby born' towards the end.

Then organize small groups of four to six people, and give each group a complete pack. Ask them to set aside the partner's cards, then share out the mother's cards so that each person has a handful, both women and men. Initially each person works independently, adding cards to the group line in the order that she or he thinks appropriate. When all cards are placed in a line, ask them to stand back and look at their line. Then ask if they want to move any cards. This promotes discussion and review, and enables people to check the information they have acquired during the course.

If you are working with couples, you can then ask the women to sit down. The labour supporters in each group can share out the partner's cards and place them alongside the mother's line to show how they might feel and respond to what is happening to her. If you are teaching women only, you can ask them to lay out the partner's cards. This gives them a glimpse of how a labour supporter might feel and react.

Once the lines are complete, ask everyone to stand or sit at one or other end of a line. This allows everyone to see all the lines. You could ask them what impression they get when looking at this line stretching ahead of them. Most people say 'it's long!'.

Your role. Once you have given the initial instructions, be available to remind people what to do, and to answer any questions. You should land up with several parallel lines, which means you could use the visual impact to show how, although there are the same number of cards in each pack, every labour is different.

If several groups are working at the same time, the end results are bound to vary. This allows you to point out the differences in the 'labours' they have laid out. For example, one line might be neatly spaced and finish sooner than the others – 'a short labour with an even pace'. Another might have big gaps between the cards between the cards at the beginning – ' a long latent phase' – or be in a wavy and disjointed line – 'a much longer labour that did not have a steady rhythm or pattern'. Sometimes one line will start well ahead of others – 'this baby was born just before 38 weeks'. Others may start much later – 'perhaps they were thinking of inducing this woman'. Some might have a gap half way down – 'perhaps this is when she went into hospital and everything stopped for a bit'. You can also reflect on the role of the labour supporter, how being there is as important as doing things – and how difficult that can be (see Chapter 13).

Situation cards

This activity helps people to consolidate what they have learned, to think about how they would act in practice, and to formulate further questions.

Timing. After the topic or topics have been covered. You could offer a selection of situation cards in one session towards the end of the course. The amount of time you need depends on the number of cards you use; allow about five minutes per card.

Optimum group size. People will benefit from discussion and sharing ideas and solutions, so groups of four to six work best.

Materials. Produce sets of four to five cards, each of which contains a situation that expectant and new parents might encounter. You could include options on the reverse of the cards to help them explore how they might deal with the situation. Include some parenting as well as labour situations. Make sure that the stories reflect the lives of the people in your classes. If you teach couples, include partners in your situation cards. If you teach single unsupported women, make sure your stories reflect their situation. Here are some samples to give you ideas.

Jo and Ben's baby is due any time now. Jo notices that her panties are feeling damp. They wonder if her waters have broken. What could she do?

- Phone the midwife or the labour ward?
- Go to hospital?
- Go the toilet, put on a dry pad and wait to see what happens?
- What else?

It is 5 am. Indira and Deepak have had a very restless night. Indira has had intermittent backache, odd contractions and general discomfort, and now the contractions have settled into a regular pattern, coming every seven minutes and lasting up to 40 seconds. She gets up to the toilet and finds she has had a show. What should they do?

- Go to hospital straight away?
- Phone the midwife or labour ward?
- Wait and see what happens?
- Go to hospital before the rush hour, which would double their journey time?
- What else?

Julie wants to have a drug-free labour. She has been having contractions for the past 11 hours and they are now really strong and close together. She is exhausted, and feels she cannot go on any longer. What could she do?

- Try changing positions? Massage?
- Ask for an epidural?
- Ask for pethidine?
- Ask for gas and oxygen?
- Ask for an internal examination to find out how far dilated she is before asking for pain relief?
- What else?

Tania is three weeks old. Sarah seems to do little else but care for her and cope with a stream of visitors. She is exhausted and upset because the flat is a mess, the washing is piling up and she hasn't had time to wash her hair. Tania is becoming increasingly fretful and is now crying a lot. Sarah is reaching the end of her tether. What could she do?

- Put a sign on the door saying mother and baby well but sleeping; do not disturb?
- Ask her visitors to do some chores for her?
- Talk to her health visitor?

- Ask a trusted friend to take the baby out for a walk so that she can rest?
- What else?

Toby is four weeks old. Recently he has been fretful and hard to pacify from about 5 pm onwards. It is 2 am and he has still not settled. Louise and Tom are both exhausted. What could they do?

- Feed and change Toby once more, then put him down and let him cry for a bit to see if he will settle?
- Take him into bed with them?
- Take him out in the car to see if that will soothe him?
- Decide that one of them should sleep while the other takes Toby into another room?
- Put Toby in a sling and walk around for a bit?
- What else?

What changes could they make to deal with this pattern?

- Make sure that Louise eats lunch and tea and rests during the afternoon so that her milk supply remains good in the afternoon and evening?
- Talk to the midwife or health visitor?
- Ask a supportive friend or relative to come in and 'dilute' the situation?
- Arrange for help with household chores?
- What else?

Marie had always wanted to breastfeed, and her partner Simon is supportive. Sam is two weeks old and a very hungry baby. Although things are going well, Marie is quite tired. Simon's mother Jane suggests that Marie might get more rest if she put Sam on the bottle. Jane says she is all in favour of breastfeeding, but that bottle-fed babies sleep for longer and it would give Marie a break if other people could feed Sam. What could Marie and James do?

- Thank Jane politely for her advice and say that all new parents are tired and that they want to cope in their own way?
- Put Sam on the bottle?
- Express some breast milk so that Jane could feed Sam occasionally?
- Ask the midwife or health visitor for support?
- Invite Jane to help with bathing or changing?
- Tell Jane she could really help if she took on some cooking and washing?
- Limit the amount of time Jane spends with them?
- What else?

Jack, who is two and a half, seems pleased with his new baby sister. Although Jack is usually contented and easy to occupy, he becomes demanding and disruptive whenever Emma feeds the baby. Emma is becoming increasingly tense about this, and it is beginning to affect the baby. What could she do?

- Save some special toys, videos or treats for feeding time only?
- Read to Jack or tell him stories while she feeds the baby?
- Enlist the help of friends to play with Jack or take him out during one or two feeds?
- What else?

Explaining the task. Ask each group to share out their cards and then take turns to read out the situation and the options. The group discusses each situation and the options. Point out that there is no absolute right or wrong, and that it is fine for people to deal with things in different ways.

Your role. You could visit each group, listen in, answer questions and add suggestions as appropriate. Once the groups have dealt with all the cards, you could invite comments and questions from the group as a whole.

Drawings

No matter what their skill in drawing, many people find this a useful way to clarify what they are thinking and feeling now and how they might feel in the future.

Optimum group size. This can be done with the whole group, any size.

Timing. This works best later in the course when people are more relaxed and confident with you and with each other. Allow around 10–15 minutes of class time.

Materials. Pencils and paper for each person.

Explaining the task. Invite everyone to do a drawing that represents, for example, how she or he is feeling about the pregnancy, how labour might be, or what life will be like with a new baby. In order for people to feel confident and safe enough to try this rather unusual way of working in the group, it is very important to stress that artistic talent is not important; neither will what they draw be commented on by anyone else. If they want to, people can each describe their own picture to their partner or to the group. It is up to you to ensure that your introductory promise is fulfilled and that nobody analyses or comments on anyone else's picture or on what they choose to say about it.

Your role. Take a back seat, but be available to ensure that nobody comments on another's drawing, and be alert to anyone who might want to talk to you.

Advert for parents of a new-born baby

This is an entertaining way to focus attention on the baby's needs and experience. It is also excellent for raising spirits and energy after covering a depressing or worrying topic.

Optimum group size. Everyone is involved, so there is no limit to numbers.

Timing. You can use this anywhere in the course; however, we usually keep it in reserve to use when spirits are low. Allow about five to ten minutes of class time.

Materials. A sheet of flip-chart paper and pen for the final brainstorm.

Process, your role and explaining the task. Invite the class to work in pairs (or fours in a couples' class) and imagine that they are an unborn baby. You could add a few words about what babies can do and what they might experience towards the end of pregnancy (see 'What babies can do' in Chapter 15). Ask them to imagine that they are about to ring the local newspaper to place an advert for the sort of parents they want. You could point out that the baby's needs will change, and that a baby, a two-year-old and a teenager require quite different skills of their parents. The task now is to focus on what they would want if they were a newborn baby. If they need a prompt, you could remind them of the scene in *Mary Poppins* where the children send notes up the chimney describing the sort of nanny they want.

Allow them a few minutes to talk, then brainstorm and chart everything they contribute. You can follow this with a discussion about meeting these needs and balancing them with the needs of the parents.

Trigger pictures

This activity can be used to promote discussion and raise new issues. It can be designed to focus on a whole variety of issues, for example, early pregnancy, labour, life after birth, older babies, toddlers and so on.

Optimum group size. This can be done with the whole group, and works best with not more than 16–20 people. You need to be present, so if you have a larger class you may need to work with a colleague.

Timing. It can be used anywhere in the course, once the group is relaxed and established. The length of time needed depends on the number of pictures you include. Allow around three to four minutes for each trigger picture.

Materials. First choose one particular aspect of childbearing – for example, early pregnancy, labour or life after birth. Make a list of the various issues that people would find useful to think about in advance. Topics for life after birth might include what a newborn baby looks like, breastfeeding, a crying baby, weighing the baby, cord care, the Guthrie test, coping with extra washing, being woken in the night, getting enough rest, sex after birth and so on. Cards for labour could show women using different positions, using gas and oxygen, in a birth pool, during an epidural Caesarean, and being monitored, and a father giving back massage or holding his baby for the first time.

This activity allows you to cover some health education issues without appearing to lecture. For example, along with pictures covering parents' concerns about early pregnancy you could include pictures of a cat litter tray, soft cheese, a glass of wine, a pregnant woman wearing a car seat belt, or a woman brushing her teeth.

Look for photos or pictures from magazines and newspapers that are likely to trigger thinking and promote discussion. Be selective. If you include too many pictures, people might get bored. Look for bright, clear drawings or photos. We suggest using around 12. Pictures from adverts can be surprisingly useful if you cut out the text. Make sure the pictures you choose reflect the cultures, ethnic groups and lifestyles that are relevant to the people in your class, and ensure that the father's perspective is specifically included. You may need to search a bit for pictures that portray parents and babies from some ethnic groups. One way of doing this is to enlist the help of your class and ask them for photos or old magazines and newspapers that are published specifically for that section of the community.

It may be difficult to find exactly what you are looking for, but while searching you may come across other pictures that could trigger issues you have not thought of. Keep an open mind, and don't limit your imagination. We have included some unlikely pictures – for example, one of a slice of rich, inviting gateau. This evokes a range of responses from 'Birth is a celebration' to 'How will I ever get my figure back?' and 'Having a baby is just a piece of cake'. Your pictures will look and last better if you mount them on stiff card and cover them with transparent sticky-backed plastic.

The process and your role. Ask the parents to draw their chairs into a circle. Spread the cards out, face down, in the centre of the circle. Invite one person to choose any card and take it back to their seat and describe what is on the card and, perhaps with the help of a person sitting nearby, to say what thoughts they have. It is very important to accept every reaction you get, even if it is quite unexpected. Then open the discussion out to include everyone before adding the key points that you think are important. Finally, suggest the card is passed around the circle so that everyone can see it while the next person is invited to pick a card. It reduces confusion if you go round the circle clockwise when asking people to pick a card, while the cards that have been discussed are passed round anti-clockwise! Repeat the process until all the cards have been discussed.

Lucky dip

This is a variation of 'Trigger pictures', and achieves much the same aim.

Optimum group size. This can be done with the whole group, and works best with not more than 16–20 people. You need to be present, so if you have a larger class you may need to work with a colleague.

Materials. Collect a variety of items that are relevant to the aspect of childbearing you want to focus on, and place them in a bag or bucket. About 8–12 items will be ample.

For example, a 'life after the birth' bag might include a breast pad, a nappy (disposable, re-usable or both), a dummy, a cord clamp, a room thermometer, and a baby-carrying sling. You could also include a pair of lacy knickers, which might start discussion about getting your figure back or sex after birth, a novel or magazine (will there ever be time to put your feet up and read?) and a clock, which could prompt questions about feeding schedules, having time to get everything done, or being woken at night.

A bag for labour could contain all the paraphernalia of a managed labour, for example a CTG trace, a scalp electrode, an epidural catheter and forceps. Alternatively, you could convey a very different message by putting in a bottle of massage oil, a music or relaxation tape, warm bedsocks, a hot water bottle, an ice pack, lip salve, a water spray and small sponge, a bath plug, a phone card and a disposable camera.

The process and your role. This is exactly the same as for 'Trigger pictures' above.

The 24-hour clock

This helps parents to realize the dramatic changes a baby makes to day-to-day routine. The strength of this activity is that people discover for themselves that life will change radically, and offers them a chance to develop strategies for prioritizing.

Timing. This works best after you have covered infant feeding, so that parents are already aware of the frequency of feeds. It takes around 10–15 minutes of class time.

Optimum group size. This can be done with the whole group, any size.

Materials. Sheets of A4 paper, with two 24-hour clocks drawn on the front and a table of five columns drawn on the back. List a range of activities in the left-hand column, including sleep as well as household chores. Make sure that your list reflects the actual lives of the people in your class. Label the next two columns 'what must be done now?' and 'what can be left now', and the final two columns 'what must be done when your baby is three weeks old' and 'what could be left when your baby is three weeks old' (see Figure 9.2 and Table 9.1). You will need enough sheets for everyone, including partners. If possible, have some spare pens and pencils available.

The process and your role. Ask everyone to fill in wedges of time that correspond with their present lifestyle. Suggest that they include cooking and other household chores, work, travel, socializing and relaxing as well as sleep. When they have completed their first clock, ask them to turn over and look at the list of activities and, using the first three columns, tick which must be done and what can be left.

Then ask them to turn back to the second clock and imagine that their baby is three weeks old. What will life be like then? Discuss how many feeds a baby is likely to need in 24 hours, and the length of time they might spend with the baby from the time they pick him or her up to the time the baby settles back to sleep. If possible, suggest they plan for at

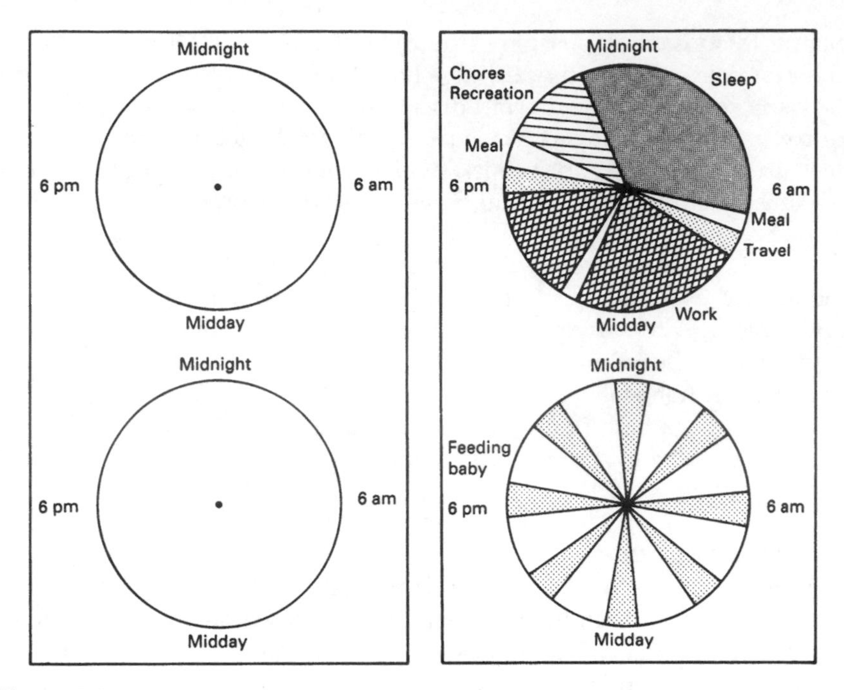

Figure 9.2

least eight or nine feeds, lasting an average of one hour each. Then ask them to put these wedges of time into their second clock. Next, if they haven't already done so, ask them to compare the two clocks – how will they fit everything in? Invite them to turn back to their priorities and see if they want to make changes. You could remind them that everything they do, including sleeping, eating, washing, cooking and shopping, has to fit into the spaces between the feeds. So they will need to be selective.

Encourage couples to talk about their priorities with each other. They may discover they are very different. If these can be raised and talked through beforehand and some compromises reached, some of the frustrations and stresses of the first few weeks of parenthood can be reduced.

Parents who insist that their life won't change that much might find it helpful to pin their clock up on the fridge. It might help them accept that there is nothing wrong with the way they are coping if life after the birth is more exhausting than they anticipated.

Buttons

This activity helps to demonstrate the subtle but profound relationship changes that the arrival of a new baby brings. For example, it might help parents to highlight sources of support and identify people who are likely to descend on them after the birth. You can suggest that, after the class, partners discuss their expectations and assumptions together so that they

Table 9.1 The 24-hour clock – setting priorities

	Now		When your baby is 3 weeks old	
	Must be done	Can be left	Must be done	Can be left
Sleeping				
Eating				
Cooking				
Washing up				
Shopping for food				
Having a bath or shower				
Washing your hair				
Bathing your baby				
Washing clothes				
Ironing				
Watching TV				
Reading a newspaper/book				
Dusting and vacuuming				
Cleaning the bathroom				
Cleaning the kitchen				
Coffee with a neighbour				
A night out with friends				
Visits from friends and family				
Buying clothes				
Aeriobics/squash/swimming				
Postnatal exercises				
Walking the dog				
DIY				
And . . .				

have a better understanding of each other's perspective and can plan more realistically.

Materials. You will need a large quantity of buttons of different shapes, sizes and colours (Figure 9.3). You can use coins instead of buttons, but some people object to putting a monetary value on themselves and their family and friends. Buttons can offer enormous variety of size, colour, shape and texture, and it is fascinating to watch the absorption and care with which people select their buttons. However, it is important to be aware that just as some people strongly dislike spiders, others dislike buttons, so it is prudent to tell people that you will use them before you tip them out. If any members of your group do have an aversion to buttons, do everything you can to ensure that they are treated with complete respect, that nobody questions or challenges them, and that they are not made to feel awkward in any way.

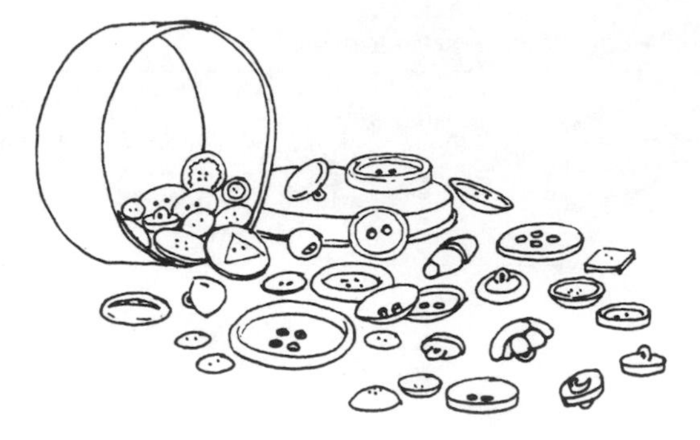

Figure 9.3

Optimum group size. Since you start by demonstrating and then everyone works individually, the only limit is the number of buttons you have!

Timing. This works best towards the end of the course, when people are comfortable and relaxed with each other and more willing to focus on life after birth. Allow around 10 minutes of class time.

The task. Individuals are invited to choose buttons to represent themselves, their families, friends and social circle, and to lay them out in a pattern that best reflects how they relate to each person and how the people relate to each other. Once the buttons are laid out, the baby can be added. Some people might alter the pattern in order to reflect the changes that they anticipate once the baby arrives.

Explaining the task. A brief demonstration is the best way to explain this activity to people. You don't need to disclose your family situation. You can lay out a couple and their friends, relatives and pets, and then add a button to represent the arrival of a baby. You may or may not want to reorganize the pattern to demonstrate how the new arrival could affect the way people interact.

It is important to stress that this is just a way of representing internal impressions so that they can be clarified and looked at. People also need to know that each time someone tries this activity it will turn out differently because the way we feel about our relationships changes. It is also important to ensure that nobody comments on or tries to interpret anyone else's pattern. This is an opportunity for personal reflection, not an invitation for others to offer their interpretations.

Then invite people to choose buttons to represent themselves and other significant people in their lives and to lay out their own family and social network as they feel it is *at this moment*. Emotionally significant friends and relatives should be included even if they live at a distance or abroad. Pets too, especially dogs and cats, should also be represented.

When they have arranged their buttons to their satisfaction, ask them to pick a button to represent their baby and place it in their pattern. Where does the baby fit into the picture? Do you need to make any changes in order to accommodate the baby? Does anyone move out? Does anyone move in? Does anyone new appear on the scene?

Your role. After the initial demonstration, you can keep an overall eye on what is happening. Ensure that nobody starts commenting on what someone else is doing, and be available in case anyone wants to talk or needs support.

Some class leaders have reservations about this activity, fearing that it could cause distress. It can certainly highlight concerns that have lain at the back of people's minds. However, the long-term benefits of identifying issues and being able to tackle or pre-empt problems can vastly outweigh temporary discomfort (see Chapters 7 and 14).

Key points

- Active learning techniques add variety and spice to a class.
- They help people to reflect and discover things for themselves.
- It is essential to give clear explanations so that parents know exactly what you would like them to do.
- Avoid tasks that have a right or wrong answer.
- The group size needs to be tailored to the activity.

References

Bligh, D. (1998). *What's the Use of Lectures?*, 3rd edn, p. 67. Intellect.

Chapter 10

Teaching physical skills

This chapter is about the principles of helping people to learn skills for coping with pregnancy, for the very physical process of giving birth, and for looking after a baby. We have called these physical skills, and there are dozens you could include in your classes.

Starting with yourself

Before deciding what to include and what to leave out, think about your own attitudes to each of various approaches you could use. If you are passionate about exercise, massage, positions for labour, relaxation or meditation, this will influence your approach and may put off the parents who do not share your enthusiasm. If on the other hand you hate the idea, or if your experience on the labour ward has convinced you that teaching relaxation and breathing is pointless, this too will filter through to the people you teach and care for. As a result they will miss out on skills that they could have found useful, not necessarily only for coping with the whole of their labour, but also for coping with the stresses and strains of daily life, a Caesarean section under epidural, and parenthood (see Chapter 11).

Alternatively, you may not know how teach physical skills. This restricts your ability to vary the pace and the type of activities you include in your classes. It makes it difficult for parents to link the information you give directly to strategies that could help them cope in practice. It also reduces your ability to offer practical support in stressful situations during labour and the early days of parenthood.

Take a moment to reflect on the following questions.

- What part does exercise, relaxation and massage play in your own life?
- How relevant do you think relaxation, breathing awareness and massage are for pregnancy? For labour? For early parenthood?
- What input and training on teaching physical skills have you received?
- What training and support would help you become confident and competent?

Establishing relevance

Parents too vary in their attitudes to physical skills. Some are already convinced of the benefits, and invest a great deal of time and energy attending classes on yoga, aquanatal exercise or tai chi, or active birth classes. Others are completely turned off by the thought of such activities. People who are reluctant to try anything physical are more likely to participate if you start by identifying how they might benefit. Make sure however that you offer carrots rather than sticks. You will find suggestions on how to do this in relation to relaxation, breathing and massage in the following chapters.

Moving from information to mastery

Information – knowing what to do – is important, but it is not enough. If parents are going to feel confident enough actually to use the skills you teach, they need to have mastered them for themselves. This means they need to try them out and practise them several times.

For instance, you might decide to teach positions for labour. One approach is to demonstrate a variety of positions and distribute a handout illustrating them. These give people the *information* that various positions are possible, but little else. If they have never tried these positions in advance, the chances that they will use them in labour when under stress, in an unfamiliar place and surrounded by strangers are virtually zero. After just one practice, use rates will still be very low.

However, if you decide that positions are important, you could include several practices in different classes, with a variety of explanations about why they are useful. You might even give 'homework', although people almost never practise between sessions even if you urge them to and enquire how they got on. With frequent opportunities to practise over time, parents get the 'feel' of that skill and make it their own.

Parents will only have the time to practise and repeat a small number of skills during your course. By prioritizing and then checking postnatally, you can discover whether or not you chose the appropriate skills. Did parents actually use what you taught? Which were particularly helpful? What skills do they wish they had covered? Their answers will help you to fine-tune your selection.

The environment

Where you teach will have a direct impact on the physical skills you can include. The job will be easier if everyone has a solid, moveable chair without arms. Group members could bring a small pillow or two to make chairs more comfortable and adapt them to various uses. A reasonably clean carpeted floor is important, as this encourages kneeling when trying out positions for relaxation or massage. If you can assure privacy and freedom from interruption, people will feel more willing to experiment.

If your room falls short of these minimal requirements, modify it if you can. Moveable screens can be used to improve privacy in a room that is overlooked. Ask, persistently if necessary, for appropriate chairs. If you are short of equipment, try approaching local voluntary groups for help. If the room is uncarpeted, try asking a local carpet merchant for off-cuts and out-of-date sample squares so that each person can have his or her own soft patch of floor. Alternatively, ask parents to bring a cushion to kneel on. Don't worry if your teaching room is small or you don't have mattresses or a large supply of pillows. Most physical skills, including relaxation, can be taught very effectively without these (see Chapters 11 and 12).

Reducing embarrassment and resistance

Most of the physical skills taught in antenatal classes are outside people's everyday experience. You may have suggested dozens of times that, with their partner's help, women try out positions for second stage. For you such a suggestion is a commonplace, but for each new group it is unusual to say the least!

Many of the skills you teach will involve parts of the body that are rarely if ever discussed in public. You may invite people to touch each other in front of others, or suggest to reluctant, tired pregnant women that they move to another position. In these and many other instances, you teach against resistance. Because of this, you need to accommodate modesty, and cajole reluctant adults to do something they would rather not do. Here are some suggestions to make this sometimes difficult task easier.

Getting people started. Once again, your attitude and expectations are crucial. So be positive, cheerful and relaxed, and above all *expect* them to participate. Gentle but persistent encouragement will usually get even the most reluctant people into action, and once started, most are willing to continue. Acknowledge and sympathize with their lethargy – 'I know you don't want to get up, but give it a try!'.

Make all your instructions optional. Once you have got people started, invite people rather than telling them what to do – 'If your arms are crossed, try resting each hand on your knees . . .'.

Start with skills that are probably safe. If you move from everyday things to the more intimate, people will begin to trust you and each other. Choose the simplest and least demanding or threatening approaches in early classes. Later in the course, people are more likely to be willing to try out things that would have felt just too risky earlier on.

Make sure you believe in the usefulness of everything you teach. Your conviction will come across to the group and increase their willingness to follow instructions.

Involve partners. If partners (or just one partner) are present, use approaches that involve them and expect them to participate. Classes should not be a spectator sport, as this is embarrassing for everyone and fails to show partners how they can be supportive and benefit from what you are teaching (see Chapters 11 and 12).

Non-participants

No matter how you approach trying out new physical skills, some people may never join in. They are free to opt out, and will have all kinds of reasons for their reluctance. Some may hold cultural or religious taboos against touching other people, against men and women touching in public, or against adopting different positions in the presence of the opposite sex. Others may find touch intrusive, find it frightening to relax amongst strangers, or become alarmed when they pay attention to their breathing. Maybe they can't imagine sitting in a group with their knees wide apart, or they are so frightened by the thought of giving birth that even pretending to do so is beyond their courage.

The only way find out for sure what stops someone having a go is to ask them. If you decide to ask, make sure you do it discreetly so that they are not further embarrassed by being put on the spot in public. Treat reluctant people with respect and include them whenever possible, but always take a relaxed approach and allow them to decide on their level of participation. If you discover, for example, that a woman is unusually distressed by the prospect of birth or that she has been abused, arrange appropriate help and support. If you think that someone in your class might find certain activities unacceptable, have a quiet word with them in advance. Explain what you will be doing, and ask how they would feel about participating.

Broadening the relevance

Including physical skills has several benefits. People tend to become more involved and lively, and the group often becomes more cohesive. At the same time, you can give them a glimpse of the pressures and feelings to come. Perhaps they are trying to relax in a room full of strangers while ignoring the workmen outside the door – tell them that labour wards can be like that, too. Other analogies abound. Women may feel tired and unsure whether they have the energy to try out different positions. However, caring for a new baby will mean doing things when they don't really want to. Discovering they can do so in your class may help them later when their baby's demands cannot be postponed. In the same way, asking couples to touch each other in public foreshadows the experience in the labour room.

For maximum effectiveness in teaching physical skills, here are some fundamental points.

- Do them often, in short bursts of five or ten minutes.
- Do them as and when they fit into the rest of the programme so that, with as many topics as possible, there is a smooth flow between information, physical skills and attitudes, and feelings. Avoid having to move rooms or change the class leader (see Chapter 18).
- Do them whenever you feel the group would benefit from a change of pace or an injection of energy.
- Do them whenever the class gets bogged down in theory or statistics. Refocus by inviting them to try out practical approaches that could help them cope with an episiotomy, an emergency Caesarean section, forceps, or a Ventouse.
- Do them often enough and in a variety of contexts so parents move from copying what they see to mastering the skill for themselves. If you do, you give parents a resource for the rest of their lives.

Key points

- Your own attitudes to physical skills influence your ability to teach them effectively.
- Parents need to understand the relevance of what you ask them to do.
- Embarrassment and resistance can be reduced if you:
  - make the environment as private and comfortable as you can
  - adopt a relaxed and positive approach
  - make your instructions optional
  - start with the least threatening activities
  - involve partners and explain how they too could benefit
  - include short sessions throughout the course.

Chapter 11

Relaxation and breathing awareness

This chapter suggests ways in which you can help people to identify unwanted tension, the ways in which unwanted tension affects them as individuals, how to release it, and how these skills can be applied to the stresses of labour and parenthood.

Why teach relaxation and breathing awareness?

The ability to release unwanted tension is a life skill that can be used in everyday situations and can benefit everyone. It is useful for managing unwanted stress and anxiety, and can improve people's feelings of confidence and control. Being able to release tension can enhance people's ability to deal with the stresses of traffic jams, job interviews, physical examinations, dental treatment, a crying baby or a rebellious toddler. It is a useful strategy for managing pain. It is also a good way of encouraging expectant and new parents to take a little time for themselves.

Why teach relaxation and breathing awareness for labour?

The overwhelming majority of women experience pain in labour. Research into pain management has highlighted a number of relevant factors.

- Pain and the anticipation of pain provoke anxiety, which results in muscle tension and leads to the release of pain-inducing substances. The result is an escalating cycle of pain–anxiety–tension (Read, 1950; Craig, 1989).
- Pain is a powerful respiratory stimulus (McDonald, 1999), and breathing inevitably alters during labour. Some women are able to 'just let go and go with the flow'. However, others become tense and panic. Teaching breathing awareness can enhance women's ability to release unwanted tension, and help them to respond flexibly to the demands of

their body and to feel in control of their behaviour. It can also be a used as a distraction technique, and can help people to maintain or regain their equilibrium in many other stressful situations.
- Pain and emotional distress increase cortisol and catecholamine levels, which can affect the length and intensity of labour (McDonald, 1999).
- Relaxation has been shown to increase people's ability to tolerate pain. Relaxation and controlled breathing can also increase their ability to deal with anxiety, and can improve feelings of control over stressful and painful experiences (Crothers, 1994; Turk and Okifuji, 1999; Weisenberg, 1999). Slade *et al.* (1993) observed that personal satisfaction is strongly associated with the ability to control panic in labour, rather than with the ability to control pain.
- Expectations of pain and stress tend to be fulfilled. People who have developed coping strategies and believe that they can manage their pain cope better than those who feel helpless. Confidence in coping strategies can influence the body's own pain-relieving and immune responses (Weisenberg, 1999).

Starting with yourself

Relaxation

Your attitudes towards relaxation will have a profound effect on what you teach and how you teach it. If you are an advocate, keep in mind those people who are turned off by the idea. You may need to temper your enthusiasm and start by helping people to identify for themselves why these skills might be useful for life as well as for labour and parenting.

If you are not convinced of the value of relaxation, try responding to the questions we suggest that you raise with parents to establish the relevance of relaxation to daily life (see below). Try out one or two of the relaxation scripts. The quick relaxation and the standing relaxation (see below) are especially useful for letting go of tension at work. Ask someone to read the script slowly while you try it out, or record the script and play it back so that you can try it out for yourself. If you are sceptical about the effectiveness of relaxation in labour, think about the experiences that underpin your attitudes. Perhaps it did not work for you. You may have been disillusioned by seeing women in labour who have been disappointed when relaxation and breathing techniques have failed to bring them as much relief as they had hoped for. If so, were people's expectations unrealistic? Relaxation and breathing techniques do not remove pain; they are a strategy for reducing and managing it. Were the women who tried to use them in labour supported in doing so? However much a woman has practised relaxation skills, it can be hard to apply them in the turmoil of labour without continuous encouragement and support, especially in a high-tech environment (Spiby *et al.*,1999; Nolan, 2000).

If you remain sceptical about the role of relaxation for labour, ask yourself: does this negate its use in other situations? Have you ever said to a pregnant, labouring or newly delivered woman, 'just relax'?

Breathing awareness

Over the years, attitudes towards teaching breathing for labour have changed dramatically. At one time, a pattern of defined breathing rates and levels was taught at most antenatal classes. This approach went out of favour when women were encouraged to follow a fixed and imposed pattern of breathing rather than respond to their own physiological needs. Reacting against this, some class leaders started to encourage women to breathe freely in response to what was happening in their bodies. Others began to ignore the issue of breathing altogether.

Many parents, however, expect to learn 'breathing'. Some may even believe that it will ensure a comfortable, easy labour. If the issue is not addressed and put into proportion, they may feel let down by the classes. Alternatively, they may continue to have unrealistic expectations and be shocked in labour when breathing does not bring the relief that they anticipated. Where do you stand on the continuum of structured to *laissez-faire* breathing? What have you read? What have you seen work? What do women say afterwards about breathing: in labour – in the first stage; at the end of first stage; in the second stage? If you have given birth, what did you find helpful or unhelpful? How will you respond to women who want to learn 'the breathing'?

If you decide that it would be helpful for women to know in advance that their breathing will alter in labour and that they will find it easier if they can 'go with the flow', you need to decide what you will do in your classes.

Who teaches these skills?

Some people believe that relaxation and breathing should only be taught by specially trained 'experts'. In reality, the ability to teach them effectively can be learned by anyone who takes the time to think through the issues and gather ideas and information, and to develop and practise these skills. The ability to teach them enhances your skills as a leader. It enables you to vary the pace and focus of your classes, and to link information with coping strategies. You can also use relaxation and breathing skills in your clinical practice, supporting a woman through a long labour, or helping a new mother to establish breastfeeding or to cope with a crying baby or a rebellious toddler.

Teaching relaxation and breathing

There is a wide variety of approaches to relaxation and breathing. We summarize a few in this chapter, and one other in the next. Relaxation and breathing are often talked about as separate skills, but in reality they are closely intertwined. It is very hard to let your breathing flow without being relaxed, and hard to relax if your breathing is tense and controlled. Linking the two, as we do in most of our examples, enables people to enhance their awareness and their ability to use both to help themselves in labour and with the day-to-day stresses of life.

We do not describe different techniques in depth, partly because there are other sources of this information, but mainly because, in order to be really familiar and at ease with a technique, you need first to have experienced it for yourself. So take every opportunity you can to participate in other people's relaxation sessions. Not only will you learn new techniques, you will also enjoy the benefits for yourself. In addition, listen to tapes and read about other people's ideas. Then, because it never rings true when a leader uses someone else's approach word for word, develop your own unique style, words and images.

You may find it helpful to practise with friends, family or colleagues. Lead them through a relaxation sequence, then ask them to tell you what they liked and what could be improved. Or you can use a tape recorder. Afterwards, listen to the tape as though it was someone else talking and identify what is good about it and what needs improving.

Incorporating relaxation and breathing awareness into the course

Frequency

How often will you include relaxation in the course? In order to acquire and develop these skills, people need plenty of practice. They also need to believe that they can use them effectively (Spiby *et al.*, 1999; Weisenberg, 1999). It is tempting to hope that everyone goes home and practises assiduously between each class. In reality, many people don't. They are more likely to benefit and develop confidence if you offer them frequent opportunities to practise during classes. This need not take up too much time. Short sessions within each class are often more effective than one or two long ones, and people who are reluctant are more likely to participate. If relaxation and breathing skills are taught in separate sessions, people who don't fancy the idea can opt out and will therefore miss out. You limit your ability to link physical skills to the topics you are discussing, and reduce the impact of what we see as the central message about relaxation: that it is a core skill and can be part of everything.

Timing

When in the class will you teach relaxation and breathing skills? If you include them in several classes, try varying the timing. In this way you can include them when you need to change the pace and atmosphere, and you can link them directly to the topics you have been discussing.

Variety

If you teach only one approach, you will please some of the people all of the time and the rest not at all. By offering variety, you are more likely to ensure that all the class members find a method that makes sense to them.

Establishing the relevance of relaxation

Acting on the assumption that teaching relaxation is 'a good thing for expectant parents to learn, so let's just get on with it', or announcing 'now we are going to do relaxation', may mean that some class members switch off. A more inviting approach is to start by helping people to consider how releasing tension can help in everyday situations. Here are some ways of doing this.

You could ask: 'What changes do you notice in your body when you are in a stressful situation? Imagine, for example, that you a late for an important meeting ... You are on a bus or in your car, stuck in a traffic jam and time is ticking by'. Group members may volunteer responses, or you may actually see people tense their shoulders and fists.

You could elicit further responses by asking: 'Where else do you tense up? What happens to your jaw muscles? To your breathing and your heart rate? Anyone get a dry mouth? Feel hot and bothered?'; 'How do you feel when you have all these physical reactions to stress? Can you think clearly? Do you arrive calm and in good shape?'; and 'What difference would it make to reduce these responses to stress?'.

You could also establish the relevance of releasing tension to managing pain. You could ask if anyone has used relaxation to manage pain, or you could invite the class to imagine being in pain. For example, 'Have you noticed what happens when you stub your toe? What's the first thing you do? Swear? Hold your toe? Tense up? Hold your breath? What else? Have you noticed that it takes a second before you actually feel pain, and you've already tensed up in anticipation? Does the tension help? Next time try breathing out and letting go'.

You could follow this with a short, simple introduction to relaxation, which offers people an opportunity to find out what it feels like to let go. Afterwards you could suggest that, during the following week, they pay attention to their physical reactions when they get angry or tense or hurt themselves. Ask them to notice where they tend to tense up first, and where the tension spreads to. Then suggest that they try letting go and notice how that feels.

With this approach, you are already linking the topics of relaxation, stress, breathing and pain. You can build on this when talking about labour and parenting in subsequent classes.

One way of establishing the relevance of relaxation to labour is to start by asking people to compare and contrast labour with a physical activity such as running a marathon (see Chapter 9). This helps people to identify for themselves the physical stresses and strains of labour, and to consider what they can do to conserve their energy and help themselves.

Some women may think that relaxation is irrelevant because they are planning to have an epidural or an elective Caesarean. You could invite them to think about how it could help in early labour, or whilst having an epidural inserted. They could practise relaxation lying down, using a sheet or pillow to simulate the screen that will be across their upper chest during the operation.

You might also suggest that relaxation is equally useful for labour partners. It is hard to remain relaxed when you are tired and worried. Labour companions also need to conserve their energy and keep as calm and relaxed as possible, both for themselves and for the woman in labour. Tension and stress are highly infectious and are easily transmitted from one person to another.

In a later class, you could invite participants to think about the relevance of relaxation to parenting. For example: 'Imagine that your baby is four weeks old. He has been waking several times each night, and you are getting more and more tired as the days pass. He has been restless and crying on and off all evening. It is 2 am, you have fed and changed him, and he is still crying and won't settle. How might you feel? Physically? Emotionally? How might releasing your tension help you/your partner? Help your baby to settle?'

Or you could lead relaxation with a visualization about life after birth (see below).

As well as discussing the benefits of relaxation and breathing, it is important to be realistic about its potential to help in labour, otherwise people will feel let down. Relaxation and breathing cannot eliminate pain; they are coping strategies that can help people to manage pain and stress and conserve energy. They can be a focus of attention and a distraction from the pain, can help reduce pain perception and enable people to tolerate it better (Crothers, 1994; Spiby *et al.*, 1993).

You could also invite the class to brainstorm the benefits of relaxation and add your own ideas. For example relaxation can:

- bring a sense of peace and well being
- improve posture
- reduce stress
- increase effectiveness at home and at work
- conserve energy
- help with insomnia

- make for safer drivers
- aid successful breastfeeding
- help to reassure distressed babies.

It is also an extremely useful skill for stressed health professionals and nervous class leaders!

Relaxation can be the central peg to which the skills and attitudes specific to labour can be attached (Figure 11.1).

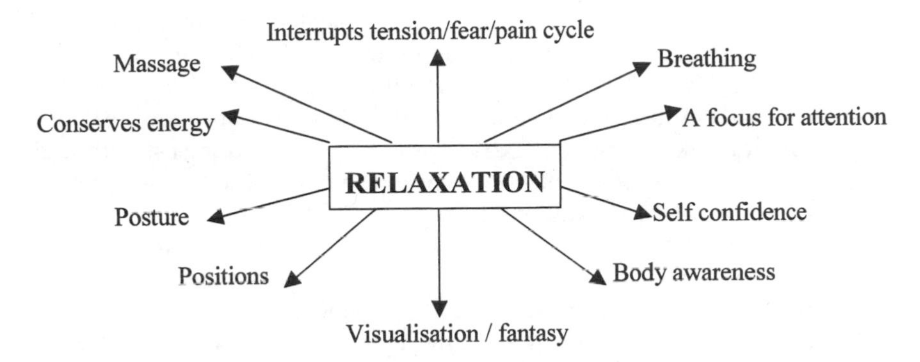

Figure 11.1

Whatever approach you use, these suggestions can help to make the sessions go well.

- Model a relaxed and unhurried approach. A brisk, business-like manner is unlikely to put people at their ease.
- Expect everyone, including partners, to join in and 'give it a try'.
- Keep sessions short, especially if you sense reluctance. It helps if you say at the beginning how long the session will last.
- In the first session, tension can be reduced by acknowledging that it is strange and perhaps difficult to come into an unfamiliar place, to be surrounded by strangers and then asked to let down one's guard and relax.
- Make sure that the room offers sufficient privacy. Feeling overlooked is inhibiting.
- Try to keep noise and interruptions to a minimum. However, if these do occur it is worth pointing out that being able to relax with activity around will be useful for everyday situations, for busy labour wards, and for parenting.
- Think about the positions you suggest that people adopt. Getting expectant parents to lie down is time consuming, and many people find it embarrassing. It can be a great position for imagining that you are walking through a forest at dawn to meet your inner self, but it fails to prepare people for the rigours of labour, which is more like being at

sea in a force 10 gale, with 10 metre waves rolling in at regular intervals. Nor does it prepare people for the stresses of daily life and parenting, most of which have to be dealt with on the hoof and not lying down in a darkened room! Invite people to practise while sitting on a chair, standing, or leaning on something or someone.

- Encourage people to get comfortable and change position if they want to. Many people feel they have to keep quite still and are too embarrassed to move despite being uncomfortable. They certainly won't learn much about relaxation in these circumstances.
- Make sure that your voice sounds relaxed. Speak clearly, and check that you can be heard by everyone. Remember that you are much more likely to go too fast than too slowly. Unless you are leading a standing relaxation, which should not last longer than a few minutes, you cannot talk too slowly! Leave pauses between phrases. Although they are familiar to you, they are new to the parents, who need time to think and act on what you are saying.
- Do the relaxation yourself at the same time (without losing the ability to lead the session!). This will help you to get the pace right.
- Choose your words carefully. Instructing people to 'relax' can be counterproductive. It may not mean anything to people who have never thought about relaxation before. Most of us have been told to 'just relax' in a tone that makes tension and irritation far more likely responses. Instead, choose everyday language and use words and phrases that actually describe the range of sensations that people can experience when they relax – for example, loose, floppy, heavy, warm, soft, let yourself sink into your chair, smooth your forehead, feel the weight of your legs against the seat of the chair, allow the chair back to support you, just let go and go with the flow.
- Giggling and laughter are ways in which people release embarrassment. If you allow them, things will work better in the long run than they would if you try to avoid or suppress them.
- Encourage people to yawn if they feel like it. It does not mean they are bored! It is an excellent way of releasing tension.
- Mention that some women may feel their babies becoming more active as they relax. By suggesting that the babies benefit and enjoy it when their mothers relax, you begin to encourage parents to see their baby as a responsive and sensitive individual.
- End the session gradually. Encourage people to start by becoming aware of their surroundings, then to move slowly and maybe stretch and yawn.
- Afterwards, invite people to review in pairs (fours in a couples' class) by asking some open questions – 'What was that like? . . . What did you enjoy . . . find helpful? . . . What was hard? . . . What did you notice about yourself?'. This will help people to think about what they experienced and, at the same time, give you some useful feedback.

Use different approaches

Choose the least threatening and most practical approaches to start with, leaving the more reflective and personal approaches until people are feeling more confident and at home with you and with each other. Choices include (starting with the least threatening, most practical approaches):

- contrasting tension with relaxation
- linking relaxation to breathing – letting go on the outward breath
- linking relaxation to posture and position
- relaxation, breathing awareness and managing pain
- quick relaxation techniques
- visualization
- touch relaxation (see Chapter 12).

Contrasting tension with relaxation

This method is good as a first introduction, especially if you choose words that really focus people's attention on the difference between relaxation and tension. It helps them to recognize what's happening in their bodies and grasp what it feels like to relax. It can be done easily and simply with people sitting on their chairs. However, some people think that asking people to tense is unhelpful, and that stretching should be used instead.

You can combine these two approaches. For example, you might begin a first session along the following lines. The dots are to remind you to go slowly.

'Turn your attention away from the room ... and towards yourself. Make yourself really comfortable on your chair ... shift about till you've got it just right ... it isn't always easy to let go in a strange environment, with people you don't really know, so take your time. Let your breathing slow down so that it is gentle and easy ... and let your breath sigh out every time you breathe out ...

Now I'm going to ask you to pay attention to various parts of your body ... to tighten or stretch them ... and then let go and notice the difference. First think about your shoulders ... pull them down towards your feet and notice where you feel the tension spread ... perhaps in the tops of your arms? Into your chest? The centre of your upper back and neck? ... Really pay attention to how it feels ... then, as you breathe out, let the tension flow out with your outward breath ... and notice how your shoulders feel ... Try it again, pull your shoulders down ... feel the tension ... notice if it spreads ... then breathe out and let go. Let your shoulders rest ... feel the difference ... Stretch your arms out in front of you ... notice how they feel, then breathe out and let them drop onto your lap and just let them rest ... Notice how they feel ... Breathe out and let them get heavier and looser.

Now think about your right leg and stretch it out – toes to nose to avoid getting cramp ... Notice how it feels ... What else tenses up? Your other leg? Your chest? ... Breathe out and let your leg drop. Feel the weight of your thigh against the chair, let your foot rest on the floor ... Now the other leg ... Try not let the first one join in ... breathe out and let it drop ... and rest. Now press your knees together, breathe out and let them fall slightly apart ... Next imagine you have a very full bladder and there is a long queue for the toilets (the gents has a queue as well!!) so you have just got to hang on! Notice what happens to the muscles between your legs ... your pelvic floor muscles. Now breathe out and let go ... let your bottom soften and sink into the chair ... breathe out and let the chair support your back ... Lastly, imagine you have a segment of lemon in your mouth ... it is extremely bitter and probably makes you screw up your mouth and eyes ... You might even notice that you also tighten your pelvic floor muscles! Now breathe out and soften your cheeks and lips, smooth your forehead.'

Afterwards, give people time to talk in small groups and invite comments and questions. You could point out how infectious tension is; how, when one part of the body is tense, other parts join in. You could then suggest that during the week they pay attention to their bodies and notice where they tense up, then try 'breathing out and letting go'.

Linking relaxation to posture and upright positions

Since most women will be mobile for part of their labour, and some will want to be upright and moving about right the way through, relaxation sessions standing up, sitting or leaning on their partners will prepare women to relax in a variety of situations. They will also reinforce the message that relaxation is useful throughout life – sitting on the bus, standing in a queue, at stressful meetings, soothing a crying baby and so on.

In order to help people to relax standing up, you need to think carefully about the instructions you give. The following is a basis for you to adapt and use in ways that are comfortable for you and appropriate for the people you teach. Unlike the others, this should be short, because pregnant women can find it hard to stand for long.

'Stand and find a space where you have room around you ... against a wall if you prefer. It's easier to do this if you take off your shoes ... you may find it better to keep your eyes open so that you don't lose your balance. Just allow your gaze to rest gently on something across the room ... Place your feet hip-width apart with your weight equally balanced, so that you have a stable base ... Notice your feet in contact with the floor ... now shift your weight gently onto your toes and rock slightly back on your heels ... shift your weight slightly onto the outside edges of your feet, and now on the inside edges ... Then find a position midway between those four ... so that you feel evenly balanced, in firm contact with the floor ... you've really got your feet on the ground! Now think about your legs ... bend your knees slightly to ensure they are not locked tightly back ... breathe out as much tension as you can from your calves and thighs, so that from your hips to your heels your legs feel loose, at ease and comfortable whilst they support you ... breathe out any tension in your buttocks ... in the muscles between your legs. Rock your pelvis gently from side to side and from front to back, circling like a belly-dancer ... now find a position where your bottom is tucked under, tummy tucked in ... and the curve in your lower back is reduced ... Let your body weight and, for the women, the weight of the baby be transmitted through your hips into your legs and down to your feet ... which are firmly in contact with the ground... Let your chest and tummy rise and fall gently and easily with your breathing ... Think about your back; imagine that you are a puppet and someone is gently pulling the string at the top of your head ... Straighten up your body, lengthen your back ... then breathe out and release the tension while retaining some of the extra height. Stand tall ... and easy. Now drop your shoulders and breathe out any tension in your arms ... let them hang loose and heavy ... stretch out your fingers and then let them go. Think about your head and neck ... Your head weighs around six pounds or 2.7 kilograms, which is a lot to carry around ... move your head gently from side to side ... look up and down, tilt it first to one side ... then the other. Now find a position midway in between in which your head is lightly balanced on your neck and shoulders ... imagine your throat getting slightly wider ... relax the muscles at the back of your neck. Let go of your jaw muscles, let your cheeks be soft and smooth, tongue resting loose in your mouth ... forehead smooth ... eyes gazing idly into the distance. Now check round your body for any tension and breathe it out ... Just enjoy the feeling.'

Relaxation and breathing awareness

This approach focuses more specifically on breathing awareness, and can be used to help people realize that they can breathe comfortably at different rates. It helps to start by putting breathing into perspective and pointing out that, like relaxation, it cannot remove pain, but it can alter the perception of pain and be a useful distraction technique. You could then point out that everyone has been breathing successfully since their birth, and that everyone adapts their breathing during exercise and manages to breathe through a whole range of painful and stressful experiences.

You can help people to realize that they naturally adapt their breathing when the circumstances demand, by asking: 'What happens to your breathing when you climb a long flight of stairs or run for a bus?'. Most will respond by saying that their breathing gets faster and shallower. Asking 'Do you have to think about changing your breathing?' makes it clear that, *if people let it*, their breathing adapts without their having to think about it.

You could then focus on issues with relevance to labour by asking, 'What happens to your breathing when you are in pain or stub your toe? ... When someone gives you a fright? ... When you are nervous or anxious?'. Most people respond by saying either that their breathing gets faster and shallower, or that they over-breathe or hold their breath. You can then point out that these are common reactions in labour, which can be handled by letting one's breathing flow and allowing it to adjust naturally as the stress of the situation demands.

Talking about breathing is not enough. People need to experiment and find out for themselves what suits them. The following points can help you to lead effective practical sessions.

- Model and encourage a relaxed, easy approach.
- Point out that each person is different and will have his or her own rate and rhythm of breathing both at rest and when under stress.
- Encourage people to release more and more tension with each outward breath, even when their breathing is quite light and rapid.
- Suggest that they pause after each outward breath, waiting until their body signals that it is time to let the next breath flow in.
- Choose your words carefully so that they create positive images – 'gentle ... flowing ... easy ... peaceful'. Avoid the word 'deep', since this tends to encourage people to take in a huge breath. Talk about slow, peaceful breathing instead.
- Use catchy, memorable phrases and imagery: 'If in doubt, breathe out'; 'If you get panicky, sigh out and let go like a balloon with a slow leak'.
- Explain how to recognize and deal with hyperventilation.
- Encourage feedback and discussion.

Some people find paying attention to their breathing is strange at first, and a few people find it difficult. This may be because they have had asthma or other breathing difficulties and associate breathing with fear and panic, or it may be because they play a brass or wind instrument or sing, and have been trained to take a very deep breath and to release it in a very slow and controlled way. The best thing for these people may be to forget about breathing and concentrate on releasing tension.

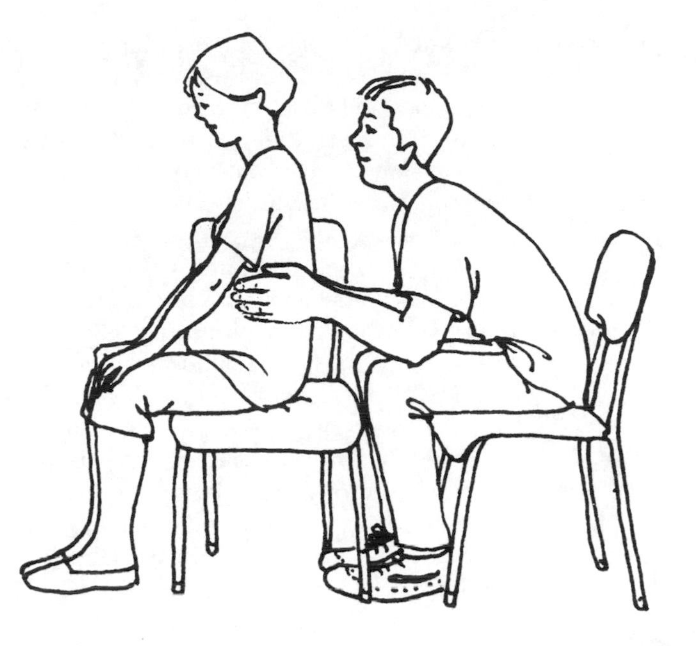

Figure 11.2

Here is one way to help parents experiment and discover what ways of breathing are available to them.

Ask people to pair up and place their chairs one in front of the other so that the person sitting behind has access to their partner's back. This means placing the front chair so the person can either sit astride it or sit with the chair back to one side (see Figure 11.2) If you are teaching couples, ask the men to sit in front and try it out first. This will help them to understand what the women are being asked to do, and gives the women an opportunity to listen and watch before trying it out themselves. Here is an example of what you might say. Try it out on friends or colleagues a few times, until you become familiar with what you want to say.

This is something that we'll do just once to help to you focus on your ability to adapt your breathing. Let's try it out. If you are sitting at the back, hold you hands palms up . . . and then place the sides of your hands on your partner's waist . . . where your partner says their waist is (or, when it is the women's turn, where her waist used to be and will be once again!). Check with your partner that your hands are in the right place . . . Now curl your hands up until your palms are in contact with your partner's sides . . . Make sure the pressure feels comfortable, no squeezing or tickling!

Now the people in front ... just let your breathing slow down ... breathe out slowly and gently ... then pause. Pay attention to your body ... and, when your body tells you it's ready, let your breath flow in down towards the hands ... and then, easily and gently, sigh out and breathe out any ... tension ... then pause until your body signals that it's time to breathe in ... let it flow in down towards the hands ... and then sigh out ... releasing any tension in your shoulders ... neck ... jaw ... And again, let your breath flow in ... pause, and sigh out ... releasing any tension around your body. Keep going, and see if you can establish a rate and rhythm that is comfortable ...

How does that feel? ... Anyone lightheaded? ... If so, slow down and take it more gently. Really pay attention to waiting until your body wants you to take the next breath in ... Slow, gentle breathing is your baseline for labour and for any other stressful event. It is calming and relaxing ... Some people use it throughout labour ... others find that as the contractions increase in intensity, they need to change the rate and rhythm just as you would if you ran up a flight of stairs.

People sitting at the back, place your hands in the middle of your partner's back ... just let them rest gently. Now, those of you in front ... just let your breath flow in, to the level of the hands, then breathe out and pause ... wait until your body wants you to breathe in again. Notice that your breathing is slightly shallower and a little bit faster ... drop your shoulders, smooth your forehead and feel yourself getting looser and floppier with every outward breath ... you can still let go on the outward breath even though your breathing is lighter. Now rest.

Those at the back ... rest your hands lightly on your partner's shoulders ... now people in front, breathe very softly and gently into the hands ... still a slight pause after each out breath, still releasing tension as you breathe out. Find a rate and rhythm that suits you ... notice that you can breathe quite comfortably at a shallower level and a more rapid rate and still remain calm and relaxed ... and rest. Now return your hands to the centre of your partner's back ... try out the middle chest breathing again ... then move your hands back to your partner's waist ... and use the slow, peaceful breathing.

Now change around so your partner gets a chance to try this out and see what it feels like.'

If you do not want to work in pairs, or you have too little time to run through this twice, you can ask the whole group to place their own hand first on their lower chest, just above their tummy; then mid-chest; and finally rest their hand very lightly on their upper chest with their thumb and first finger gently circling their neck.

Practise contractions

Having established that it is possible to breathe at different rates, you need to offer parents an opportunity to discover how to use these techniques in response to discomfort and pain. There are several approaches you can use. None of them replicates the pain of a strong contraction, but they can help people to realize that relaxation and breathing awareness can increase their ability to cope. Unless they have experienced this for themselves, they re unlikely to use them in labour.

Class leaders use a variety of approaches to practise contractions and you will probably prefer some to others. However it is important to offer parents more than one approach, as most people find some more helpful than others. You could:

- ask parents to lean against a wall, with their shoulder blades and lower back in contact with the wall and feet firmly on the floor, about hip width apart. Then ask them to slide down a little until their knees are flexed, *then hold the position* and, as the discomfort in their legs builds up, to use relaxation and slow breathing and see if they hold the position for one minute. If the sensation gets too uncomfortable, suggest that they let their breathing become lighter and faster while continuing to 'let go' on each outward breath (see Figure 11.3). It helps if you demonstrate the position first, ask women wearing heeled shoes to take them off so that their feet are firmly on the ground, *and ensure that nobody stands against doors, cupboards or anything that might not support them.*
- invite parents to kneel down with a chair next to them for balance, and then, keeping their back straight, drop their bottom onto their heels. Once you are sure that everyone is keeping their back straight, ask them to repeat the movement, but stop half way and then hold it and breathe and relax for up to one minute. Most people find this more stressful, and need to move from slow to shallow breathing to cope with the discomfort (see Figure 11.4).
- ask parents to use relaxation and breathing awareness while you talk them through a contraction, say 40 or 50 seconds long. Describe the contraction and how it might feel, and what partners might be doing. As the contraction intensifies, gradually raise your voice until you are speaking very loudly at the height of the contraction – and let it quieten again as the contraction fades.
- possibly suggest that people give each other Chinese burns or pinch each other. These can work well, but need to be used with caution, especially if you suspect that anyone in your class is being dominated or abused by their partner. An alternative is to ask women to relax and breathe through the discomfort of having their arm compressed by a blood pressure cuff.

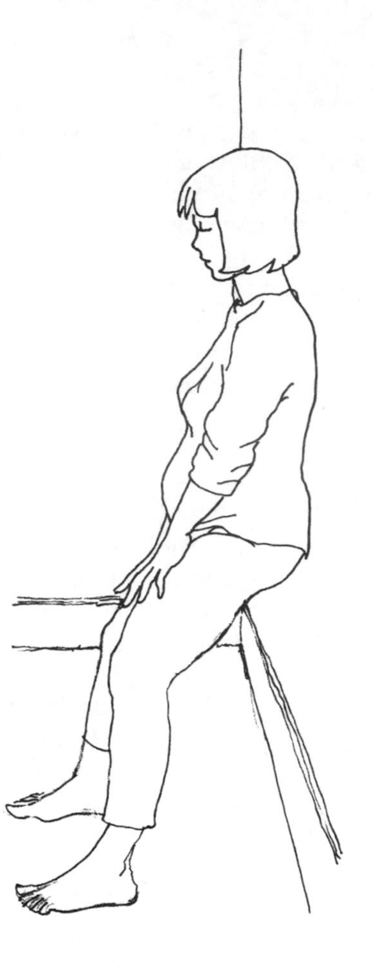

Figure 11.3

Transition and second stage

As well as teaching breathing as a pain and stress management strategy for the first stage, you might want to include discussion and practice for coping with an anterior lip and with pushing.

Coping with an anterior lip. This is one of the few occasions when the message 'just let go and go with the flow' may not apply, so it is vital that women understand why they might be asked to wait a little longer before pushing strongly. They also need to try out appropriate positions, for example all fours with the head lower than the hips. Some (but not all) leaders advocate teaching specific breathing patterns to avoid or minimize pushing, for example light and rhythmic breathing or panting. Brayshaw and Wright (1996) suggest using a rhythmic pattern of three on each outward breath – 'puff–puff–blow'.

Pushing. Since there is no evidence to support directed pushing in the second stage, and some evidence to indicate that it may be harmful (Caldreyo-Barcia, 1979; Thomson, 1988; Enkin *et al.*, 2000), you may

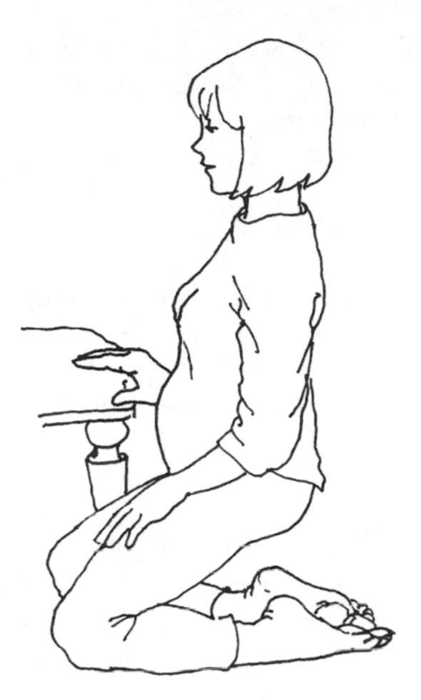

Figure 11.4

need to counterbalance media images of women being exhorted to push till they are blue in the face. Instead you could encourage them to choose and practise upright or forward leaning positions, to move freely and respond to their own urges to push (Walsh, 2000). You might also point out the importance of relaxing the pelvic floor and the mouth, as tension in one tends to be mirrored in the other!

Quick relaxation techniques

In stressful situations – during a busy working day, at the beginning of each labour contraction, or when the baby fills her nappy just after being changed – people need to be able to release unwanted tension very quickly. Having established some awareness and skill by using the techniques we have covered so far, you can introduce a variety of methods that will help people to reduce tension at will. The first consists of three simple actions:

- Think STOP
- Push your shoulders DOWN
- Breathe OUT long and deliberately, letting all the tension flow out with the outward breath.

The relaxation ripple consists of releasing tension from the top of the head to the tips of the toes in one continuous wave. As an introduction, ask people to tense up all over, then to release the tension with a long, slow breath out, relaxing from the top of the body down to the toes in the space of that outward breath. Having practised this once or twice, people should not tense up to start with, but should continue to practise simply letting go from head to toe with one long, releasing breath out.

Visualization

There is an infinite variety of visualization techniques you can use with people who have begun to develop some skill in relaxation. Before you decide to use visualization, think through what you are trying to achieve and then devise your own script, using words and phrases that you are comfortable with and are appropriate to the people you teach. Here are a couple of examples.

Thinking about your baby

This exercise can help parents get in touch with their baby very early in the antenatal course and recognize that he or she is already a sensitive individual. Having completed a relaxation session with people in comfortable positions (not standing up!), you can invite people to do the following with you.

> '... turn your attention towards your baby ... imagine him or her, curled up inside, safe, warm and comfortable ... constantly held ... always at the right temperature ... rocked by the mother's movements. Your baby is already able to hear, is already familiar with the sounds within the mother's body ... with the rhythms of her heart, her breathing and the way she moves ... He or she is also familiar with the rhythms and cadences of the mother's voice and the voices of those close to her ... If they have heard their father's voice before birth, newborn babies can recognize his as well as their mother's voice ... Your baby can already dimly perceive light ... can suck his or her thumb ... swallow and pee. He or she may already have recognizable times for rest and activity ... or be specially prone to hiccoughs ... Just spend a few minutes with your baby, who is growing and preparing for the birth, just as you are ... Then, in your own time, turn your attention back towards your body ... and to the room ... take your time. Remember that you can go back and spend time with your baby whenever you choose.'

This exercise conveys a lot of information about what the baby is like and can do in a way that includes the parents. Notice that the words are chosen with care to include fathers. If you talk about 'your uterus', he is left out. Many people find this exercise an emotional experience, and a few (usually women who already have children) will cry afterwards.

When they talk about why they reacted in this way, they often say they realize how little time and attention they have given their growing baby because the demands of the child/children they already have are so constant. It usually helps if you encourage them to notice that they have now spent time with the new baby. You could also acknowledge that being pregnant and parenting small children at the same time is extremely demanding, and that they are doing their very best under difficult circumstances.

The shopping trip

This exercise is useful towards the end of the course, when people are familiar with relaxation and have already begun to think beyond the birth to being parents. You could use words like these.

> 'Sit comfortably, either in a chair or well propped up with cushions, and find something – a pillow, a folded jumper or a handbag – to hold as if it is your baby. Place the 'baby' on your chest so that he or she can hear your heartbeat and feel the rhythm of your breathing. Hold him or her gently but securely ... Imagine that your baby is three weeks old. You have just come back from shopping ... you are tired ... you didn't get much sleep last night ... You have several bags of shopping to put away ... the kitchen is a bit of a tip ... and you are anxious to get on, tidy it up and get the evening meal. Your baby is restless and unsettled, even though the last feed was less than an hour ago. Take a decision to leave the shopping and the mess ... It will wait. Settle yourself comfortably with your baby ... hold him or her close to you ... slow your breathing ... and with each outward breath, release the tension in your shoulders ... your neck ... let your head rest or find a position in which it is easily and effortlessly balanced on your neck and shoulders. Breathe out the tension in your jaw and cheeks ... smooth out your forehead. Let your arms be soft, welcoming and supportive as you gently cradle your baby. Let your chest and tummy rise and fall peacefully as you breathe ... Allow your back to sink into the supports ... let go of your legs from your hips to your heels. Just take time to rest ... warm, safe, protected and protecting ... enjoy the feeling of your baby snuggled against you ... the softness, warmth and smell of his or her skin. Feel the movements he or she makes ... As you relax and feel peaceful, your baby, who is very sensitive to your moods and feelings, is likely to do so too. Then, when you have rested ... gently stretch and move ... and slowly prepare to get on with whatever needs to be done.'

It helps if you model a good position in which to sit and hold the 'baby'. It is more graphic if you use a realistic doll to demonstrate this (see Figure 11.5).

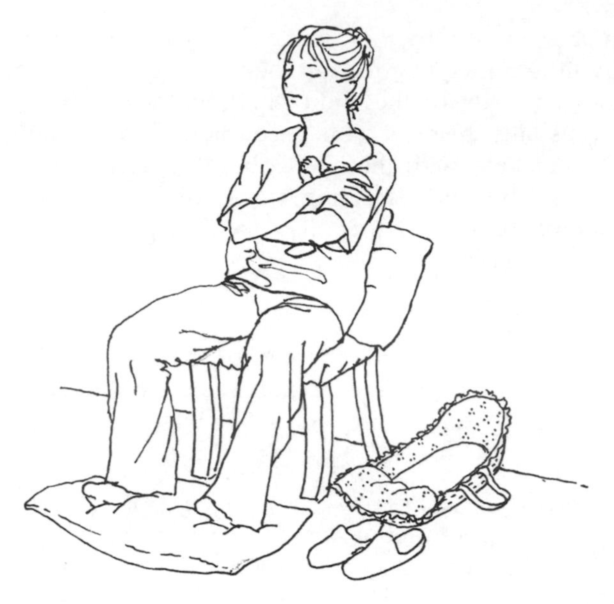

Figure 11.5

Key points

- Relaxation and breathing awareness are life skills that can benefit everyone.
- There are both physical and psychological reasons for teaching relaxation and breathing awareness for labour.
- Your own attitudes will have a strong influence on your ability to teach effectively.
- Relaxation and breathing awareness can be taught by anyone who uses it themselves and takes the time to develop their skills.
- It is important to establish relevance before teaching relaxation and breathing awareness.
- Frequent short sessions throughout the course are likely to be more effective than fewer long ones.
- Offering a variety of approaches maintains interest and increases the likelihood of everyone finding one that appeals to them.

References

Brayshaw, E. and Wright, P. (1996). *Relaxation and Exercise for the Childbearing Year*, pp. 33–4 Haigh and Hochland Publications Ltd, in conjunction with the Royal College of Midwives.

Caldreyo-Barcia, R. (1979). The influence of maternal bearing-down efforts during the second stage on fetal well-being. *Birth and the Family Journal*, **6**(1), 17–21.

Craig, K. D. (1989). Emotional aspects of pain. In: *Textbook of Pain*, 3rd edn (P. D. Wall and R. Melzack, eds), pp. 220–30. Churchill Livingstone.

Crothers, J. (1994). Labour pains: a study of pain control mechanisms during labour. *Journal of the Association of Chartered Physiotherapists in Obstetrics and Gynaecology*, **74**, 4–8.

Enkin, M., Keirse, M. J. N. C., Neilson, J. *et al.* (2000). *A Guide to Effective Care in Pregnancy and Childbirth*, 3rd edn, p. 297. Oxford University Press.

McDonald, J. S. (1999). Obstetric pain. In: *Textbook of Pain*, 4th edn (P. D. Wall and R. Melzack, eds), pp. 661–87. Churchill Livingstone.

Nolan, M. (2000).The influence of antenatal classes on pain relief in labour. 2: The research. *The Practising Midwife*, **3**(6), 26–31.

Read, G. D. (1950). *Childbirth without Fear*, p. 21. Heinemann.

Slade, P., MacPherson, S. A., Hume, A. and Maresh, M. (1993). Expectations, experiences and satisfaction with labour. *British Journal of Clinical Psychology*, **32**(4), 469–83.

Spiby, H., Henderson, B., Slade, P. *et al.* (1999). Strategies for coping with labour: does antenatal education translate into practice? *Journal of Advanced Nursing*, **29**(2), 388–94.

Thomson, A. M. (1988). Management of the woman in normal second stage of labour, a review. *Midwifery*, **4**, 77–85.

Turk, D. and Okifuji, A. (1999). A cognitive-behavioural approach to pain management. In: *Textbook of Pain*, 4th edn (P. D. Wall and R. Melzack, eds), pp. 1431–43. Churchill Livingstone.

Walsh, D. (2000). Part six: Limits on pushing and time in the second stage. *British Journal of Midwifery*, **8**(10), 604–8.

Weisenberg, M.(1999). Cognitive aspects of pain. In: *Textbook of Pain*, 4th edn (P. D. Wall and R. Melzack, eds), pp. 345–58. Churchill Livingstone.

Chapter 12

Positions, massage and exercise

This chapter outlines some principles to consider when teaching positions, massage and exercise, and suggests a few approaches. It is not comprehensive, since each of these topics merits a book of its own and there are many other sources of information.

Teaching positions

Why teach positions?

Upright postures and mobility in the first stage of labour have been shown to increase the efficiency of contractions and reduce the need for pharmacological pain relief. They also shorten the second stage, and reduce episodes of severe pain (Enkin *et al.*, 2000, pp. 263–4, 291). In addition, many women feel more in charge and better, both emotionally and physically, if their head is literally as well as metaphorically above their uterus. Most women will be upright and mobile for at least part of their labour, and, depending on their choice and the views of their attendants, a number remain so right the way through.

Experimenting with different positions can also ease the discomfort of pregnancy. Pregnant women need to find new ways of doing everyday things. Practical tasks such as cleaning a bath and making a bed become more difficult. Later on, getting out of an armchair and getting comfortable in bed can be a challenge. By helping people to discover a variety of positions and offering them opportunities to link these with relaxation, you equip them to adapt during pregnancy and respond flexibly during labour.

Starting with yourself

As usual, your own experience and attitudes are important. How do you feel about women being active and mobile throughout labour? Do you think it unnecessary? Is it too inconvenient for those trying to monitor the baby and care for the mother? Is mobility in labour encouraged in your unit, or are your colleagues going to object if you encourage women to be mobile? What benefits have you seen or experienced? What do women who have remained mobile throughout labour tell you?

Establishing relevance

This can be done in several ways. For example, you could summarize research findings and use the activity 'Finding out about the pelvis' (see Chapter 8) to enable parents to discover the benefits for themselves. You can also use a chart, showing a cross-section of a pregnant woman at term. Start off holding the chart so that the woman is supine. Show how the mobility of the sacrum is lost in this position, and explain how the weight of the uterus presses on the mothers' main blood vessels. Now rotate the chart so that the mother is propped up, then upright, and finally on all fours, so that parents can see for themselves what a difference positions can make. You can also illustrate the benefits of gravity.

Practical approaches

Here are some key points for teaching positions in labour.

- Keep your information giving short, and spend the maximum amount of time on practising.
- Suggest that people wear loose, comfortable clothing to classes, and do the same yourself.
- Use a relaxed, casual approach when demonstrating.
- Be determined and persuasive about getting people going. Acknowledge their reluctance or lethargy, but keep up some cheerful encouragement until they move. If they don't practise in class, they are less likely to use different positions in labour.
- Invite people to try out and practise a whole variety of positions. What they like and dislike now may not apply in labour. What suits the early first stage may not work later on in the labour.
- Encourage parents to keep trying new positions in labour. Just as turning over into a new position during a sleepless night can help, changing positions during labour can in itself make things more tolerable.
- Build in opportunities for practise throughout the course.
- Link practising positions to relaxation, breathing awareness or massage.
- Encourage people to experiment at home. Which bits of furniture are the right height to lean on during contractions (see Figure 12.3)? Do they have a chair on which they could sit astride (see Figure 12.2)? How could they get comfortable on the car journey to hospital?
- Discuss ways of adapting the labour room. The fact that it contains a

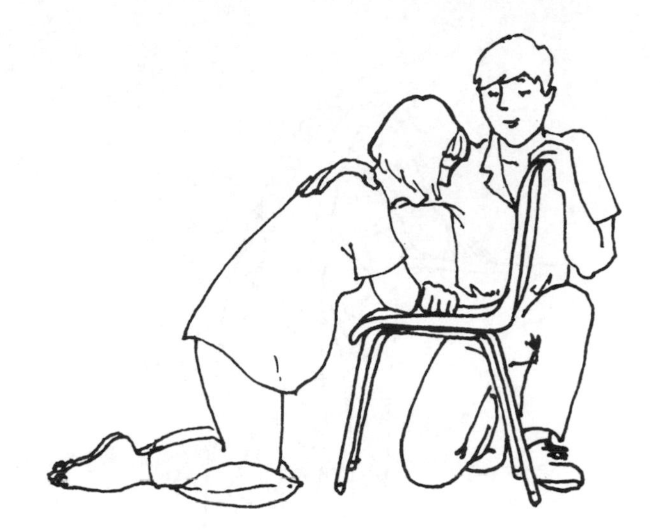

Figure 12.1

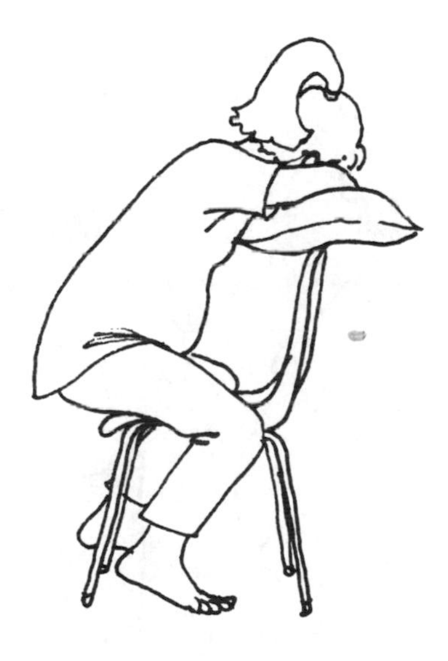

Figure 12.2

bed does not mean that the woman has to lie on it. Furniture can be moved to create space, and parents might like to bring in items like cushions or a beanbag from home.

- If you are teaching couples, encourage the fathers to help the women get comfortable in a variety of positions.

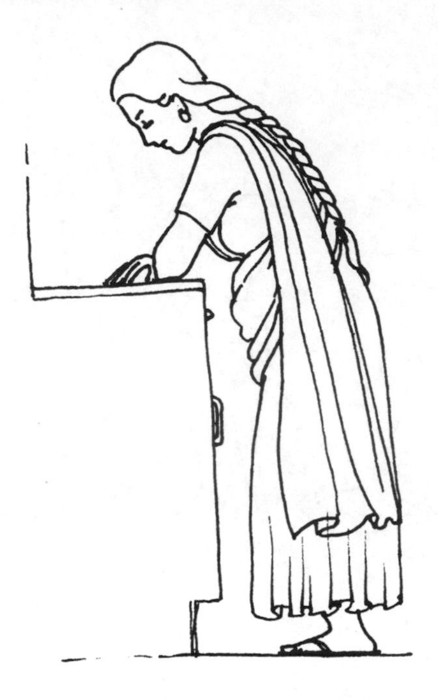

Figure 12.3

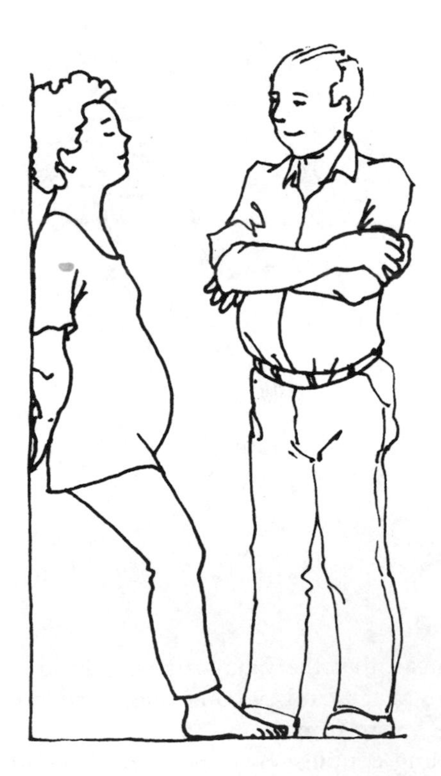

Figure 12.4

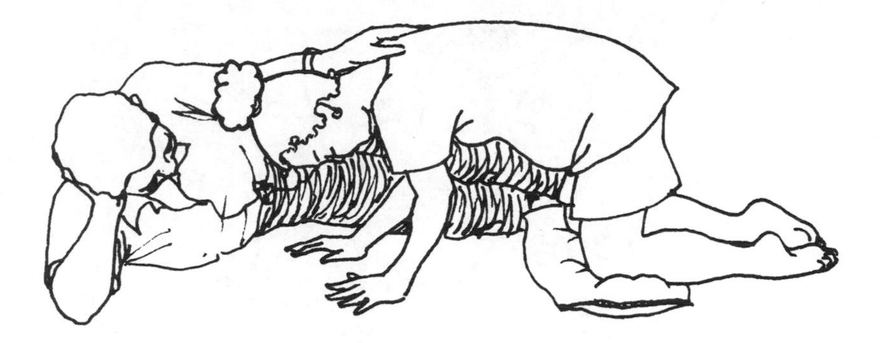

Figure 12.5

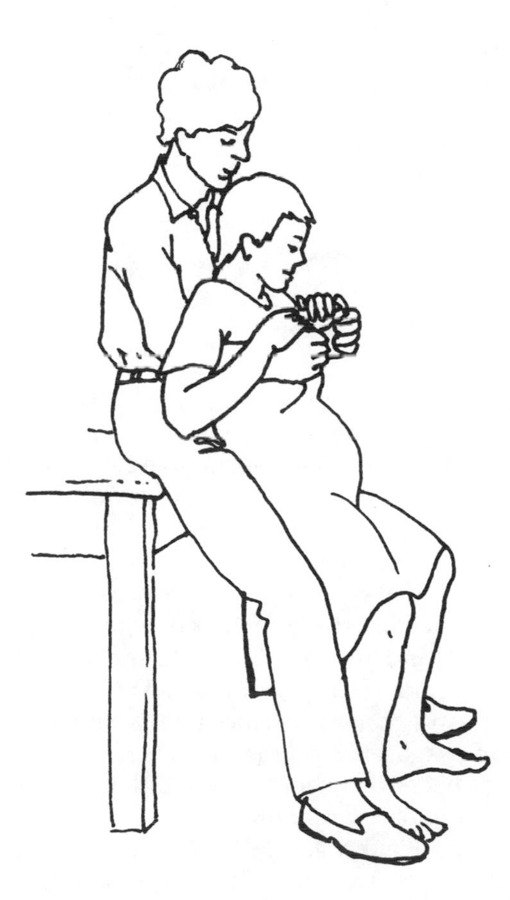

Figure 12.6

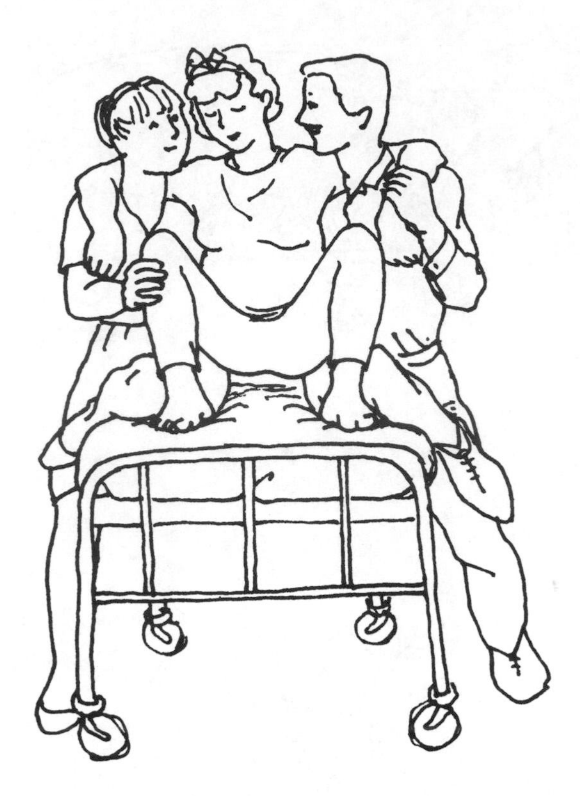

Figure 12.7

Teaching massage

Why teach massage?

Touch can be comforting. It can ease the physical and emotional stresses of everyday life, and the aches and pains of pregnancy and labour. Touching helps couples to express affection and communicate with each other and with their baby once he or she is born. Including touch and massage in your classes gives women opportunities to learn how to relax whilst they are being touched and whilst there is activity going on around them – something that will be part of their experience in labour.

A National Birthday Trust study of 10,000 women found that some 90 per cent of women found relaxation and massage good for pain relief (Findley and Chamberlain, 1999). Two small studies indicate that massage can benefit pregnant and labouring women. The women who received regular massage during pregnancy were less anxious, had less back pain, and slept better than women who did not receive massage. The massage group also had fewer complications in labour and decreased stress hormone levels. (Field *et al.*, 1999). Women who received massage in labour experienced less anxiety, less pain, and had significantly shorter labours (Field *et al.*, 1997).

Starting with yourself

Individual leaders vary enormously in what they think useful and appropriate when it comes to massage. Many are hesitant and self-conscious about it, which is surprising considering the intimate ways in which midwives in particular touch their clients. However, health professionals are trained to touch in ritualized ways and with a degree of detachment. There are good reasons for this, and it works well for many procedures. However, therapeutic touch – that is, touch that helps the other person to feel better – requires greater involvement of the person doing the touching.

How do you feel about touching and being touched? Have you ever had a massage? If not, would you consider having one? How do you feel about teaching massage? If inexperience is a factor for you, find someone who is confident. There are a growing number of health professionals and others who have done massage and aromatherapy courses. Ask them to show you what they do, and find out what it feels like to be on the receiving end. If you can, go to a workshop or study day on massage. Then reconsider what you will include in your course.

Establishing relevance

You can link touch and massage to discussion on relieving aches, pains and stress, and suggest it as another approach to relaxation (see below) or as something that babies appreciate. Make sure you mention that, however much a woman enjoys massage, there may come a time during labour when she cannot bear to be touched.

Practical approaches

There are many different ways in which you can encourage aware, helpful touch and massage in an antenatal course. You could link it to relaxation, and teach self-massage, strong back or thigh massage, perineal massage, effleurage, foot massage or baby massage.

Whatever type of massage you teach, the following can help to make the session go well.

- However sensitively you approach massage, expect some self-consciousness and embarrassment. Our society conditions many of us (and men in particular) to believe that touch is only relevant as a precursor to sex, so touching in public will seem odd. It helps if you talk about 'touch' rather than 'massage', which for some people has a rather dubious reputation.
- Be sensitive to individual needs. Touching in public may be unacceptable to some people on religious or cultural grounds. Others may find touch difficult, especially if in the past they have been touched in ways

that were not for their benefit. Make it easy for people to participate to the degree to which they feel comfortable.

- Plan when to include touch. It will probably work best once the group is well established.
- Make sure that everyone has someone to work with. If you are teaching couples, *ensure that the men receive first*. This is not what people expect, but it works well for several reasons; on the whole, women are less self-conscious about using touch in public than men, and men who have experienced the benefits are more motivated to do it well for their partners.
- Explain that this is an opportunity to find out what each person likes; nobody should put up with something that they find uncomfortable. Encourage partners to talk to each other. They cannot guess what the other person likes or dislikes.
- Encourage recipients to tell their partner what feels good rather than criticizing. For example, 'It feels wonderfully relaxing on my legs, and it would be great if you could use more pressure over my feet'. This confirms the skills of the person doing the touching, and offers them constructive information for improvement.
- Show people, step by step, what you want them to try. Ask before you demonstrate on anyone, and model a relaxed, confident approach, which focuses on and completely respects the person you are touching.
- Suggest that the touchers shake out their hands so they are loose and floppy and can mould to the shape of the part they are touching.
- Make sure that the people doing the massage are comfortable. This is a good time to point out that being a labour companion is tiring, and that partners need to conserve their energy too! Keep an eye out for anyone giving massage in a way that could cause back strain.
- Don't be put off by laughter and giggling. These are good ways for people to release their embarrassment. Remind them that everyone in the room is concentrating on what they are doing and nobody is being watched.
- Instead of telling parents they are doing something wrong, demonstrate an alternative and support them in trying it out.
- Afterwards, ask the group to review the experience. What did they like? What might be useful in labour? In everyday life? When they or their partners are tired or stressed? What do they think their baby might enjoy?

Touch relaxation

There are many ways to teach touch and massage. Here is a sample of what you might say that keeps embarrassment to the minimum and gently eases people in. It is quite detailed, so you will probably find it helpful to take it in stages, go through it several times and try it out with colleagues before using it with a class. If you have not used touch or massage in your classes before you might use just one or two stages until you gain confidence, but make sure that everyone has a turn to give and to receive. You can minimize reluctance by introducing it as just 'another way of relaxing', rather than announcing that the participants will be using touch and massage.

Stage one

'Pair up with another person, with one of you (the partner if it is a couples' class) sitting on a chair and the other (the woman) standing behind. Make sure that there is plenty of room to move around between the chairs. The people standing are going to help their partner to release tension.

This is something that you *might* use in labour, and it is a great way of helping each other to unwind after a stressful day and for soothing tense and fretful babies. I expect lots of chat and discussion during this. You cannot guess what your partner finds helpful, so ask. This is not about putting up with something that you don't like, so do tell your partner what you prefer.

People standing, place your feet about hip-width apart. If you are very tall, you might be more comfortable sitting down. Shake your hands to loosen them. Now place them on your partner's shoulders, over the muscle, not over the bony bits. Make sure your thumbs are parallel to your fingers (not sticking out at right angles), and that the whole of your hands, from your wrists to your fingertips, are resting on their shoulders. Find out how much pressure your partner likes. Now take your hands off. (See Figure 12.8).

People sitting ... next time you feel your partner's hands on your shoulders, imagine that she is absorbing all your tension ... as you feel the hands go on, breathe out and let go.

People standing, give your hands another shake, now place them back on the shoulders with the pressure your partner likes, and hold it for a few seconds.

Now, smooth your hands across your partner's shoulders and down the upper arms, as far as you can reach without bending your back. Sweep your hands off their arms rather than stopping suddenly. Imagine that you are brushing your partner's tension away. Find out if your partner finds this helpful. If not, go back to resting your hands on the shoulders.

You are in a good position to use your thumbs to release tension in your partner's shoulders. Rest your fingertips lightly on the shoulders. Press your thumbs into the muscle across the back of the shoulder – you may be able to feel the tension, or your partner will tell you where to apply the pressure. Now, keeping your thumb tips in contact with your partner's skin, use firm circular motions, moving the skin over the underlying muscle. You can also do firm circles either side of the

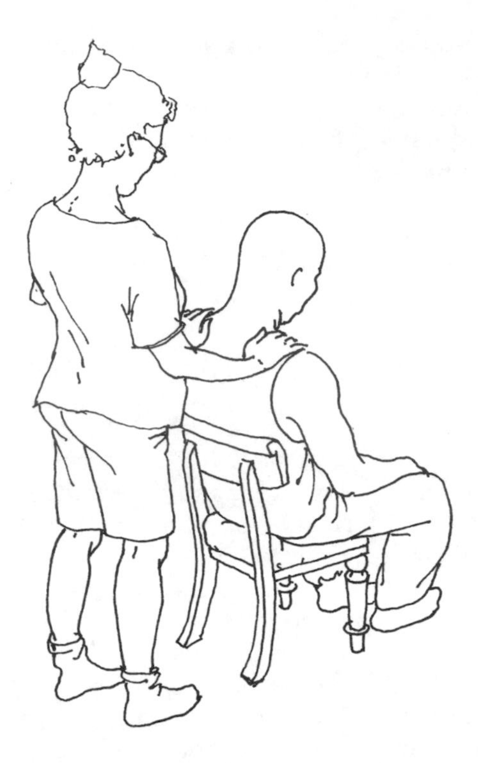

Figure 12.8

backbone. After four or five circles, move your thumbs down a couple of centimetres and repeat, then another couple of centimetres . . . and so on. Find out what your partner prefers.'

Stage two

'People sitting, turn and either sit astride your chair, or sit on it sideways so that your partner can reach your back.

Partners, kneel (or sit if kneeling is difficult) behind and place your hands back on the shoulders, then sweep them firmly down the back either side of the backbone. When you reach the lower back, point your fingers out sideways so that you can let your stroke flow off. Repeat a few times. As an alternative, you can place one hand over the backbone, fingers towards the base of the neck, and sweep your hand slowly and *gently* down to the base of your partner's back. Before you take this hand off, place your second hand at the top so that you have continual contact, with one hand sweeping down followed by the other. Find out which your partner prefers.

Now you can try firm, circular massage over the lower back, using the heel of your hand – your partner will tell you where it feels best.' (See Figure 12.9).

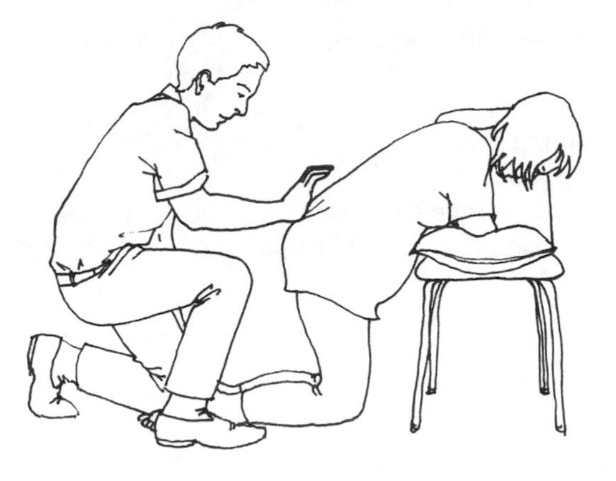

Figure 12.9

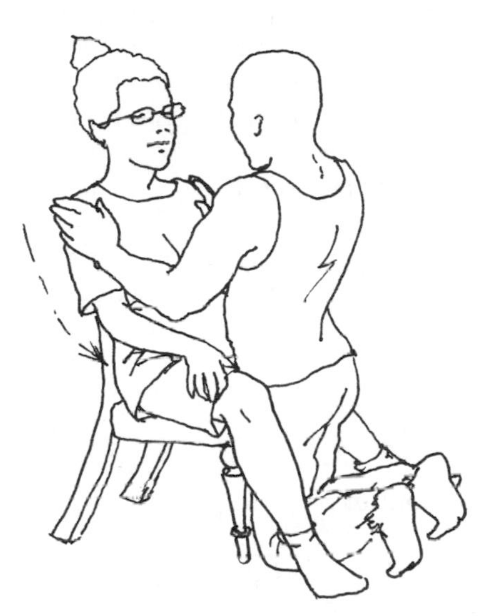

Figure 12.10

Stage three

'People sitting, turn round and sit back on your chair, with your hands on your lap and feet on the floor. Partners kneel alongside and place both hands on the shoulders, and firmly stroke across the shoulders, all the way down the arms and off your partner's fingertips.(Figure 12.10).

Now move back and place your hands firmly on the outsides of the lower thighs, just above the knees. This time, sweep your hands very firmly down the legs, running your fingers over the calf muscles at the back. When you reach the feet, circle your partner's ankles with your thumb and first finger and press down very firmly, using the heels of your hands over the centre of the feet. Hold for a few seconds and then slowly release. Now change over, it's your partner's turn.'

After a massage session, the group is usually relaxed and ready to receive some information or engage in real discussion. You could suggest that touch is a lovely way to show each other affection without having sex – which is something that may not be welcomed by some women towards the end of pregnancy or in the early days after the birth. You can also point out that babies love to be stroked, and that by practising with each other they are learning a skill that their baby will very much appreciate.

Including exercise

General exercise helps to maintain fitness. There are no proven advantages or disadvantages of exercise in pregnancy (Enkin *et al.*, 2000). Women who regularly take exercise will probably want to continue throughout pregnancy, and may already be attending active birth, yoga, aquanatal or keep-fit sessions for pregnant women. Those who do not may be willing to try a few exercises in your classes, especially if they can see why these might be useful.

There are a whole variety of exercises that you could use in your classes. Most of the books and pamphlets aimed at pregnant women mention the importance of good posture and exercise. Some go into detail about how to prepare for labour. Nearly all advocate regular exercise for the pelvic floor.

Starting with yourself

How do you feel about exercise in general and about exercises for pregnancy and afterwards? Are you keen or reluctant to exercise? Which exercises are essential for pregnant women? Do you feel confident about teaching them? If not, where could you get the information and skills that you need to include in your classes? You could contact your local physiotherapy department, attend workshops, and have a look at books and leaflets on exercise in pregnancy, including those written for parents.

Practical approaches

If you teach active birth or aquanatal classes, there is plenty of time to focus on the physical. However, in a course that balances information sharing, attitudes and feelings and physical skills, there will be limited time. You need to evaluate the evidence and decide which exercises will be most beneficial and make the best use of the time available. We suggest, as a basic minimum, pelvic floor exercises and pelvic rocking, partly because they have the added advantage of jiggling the inhibitions as much as exercising the muscles themselves! You might also want to spend a little time on posture and lifting – although avoiding and easing backache may sound more appealing!

Pelvic floor exercises

Many reasons are given for teaching and practising pelvic floor exercises, not all of which are proven. Noble (1995) cites 13. Sleep and Grant (1987) found that pelvic floor exercises did not reduce the incidence of urinary and faecal incontinence. However, they did find that women who followed an intensive programme of pelvic floor exercises reported less perineal pain three months after the birth than those who did not. While some people may doubt the usefulness of pelvic floor exercises in pregnancy, there are still many passionate advocates who believe that doing pelvic floor exercises before birth increases strength and flexibility, increases awareness (enabling women to relax the pelvic floor during the second stage), and makes it easier to do them afterwards.

If you include pelvic floor exercises, it is best to begin early in the course. You can help women to identify their pelvic floor muscles when they are finding out about the pelvis (see Chapter 8) or by imagining that they have a full bladder and there is a queue for the toilet (see Chapter 11). Alternatively, ask them to blow sharply into a fist. This usually produces a kick in the appropriate place. There are several ways to teach pelvic floor exercises. For example, you can compare the pelvic floor to a lift, stopping at each floor on the way up and on the way down; and suggest women try them during sexual intercourse. You could suggest they see if they can stop the flow of urine midstream. However, this method should only be used occasionally as a way of assessing their ability, and not as a way of practising (Kitzinger, 1997; The National Childbirth Trust, 2000).

Most people have a hard time remembering to practise and will need frequent reminders. Little and often usually works best. You could suggest women remember to practise by linking pelvic floor exercise to everyday activities such as standing in a queue, waiting for someone to answer the telephone, or brushing their teeth.

Pelvic rocking and circling are good ways to get women moving about and trying things out. They are useful for promoting physical and psychological flexibility, and can help to relieve backache during pregnancy in labour. You could point out that pelvic rocking and circling can sometimes help the baby's passage through the pelvis (Sutton, 2000). Pelvic rocking is also an ideal way to give the group a five-minute energy boost. Use it when you feel the group needs to move, get their circulation going, or recover from a gloomy discussion.

References

Enkin, M., Keirse, J. B. C., Neilson, J. *et al.* (2000). *A Guide to Effective Care in Pregnancy and Childbirth*, 3rd edn. Oxford University Press.

Field, T., Hernandez-Reif, M., Taylor, S. *et al.* (1997). Labour pain is reduced by massage therapy. *Journal of Psychosomatic Obstetrics and Gynaecology*, **18**(4), 286–91.

Field, T., Hernandez-Reif, M., Hart, S. *et al.* (1999). Pregnant women benefit from massage therapy. *Journal of Psychosomatic Obstetrics and Gynaecology*, **20**, 31–8.

Findley, I. and Chamberlain, G. (1999). ABC of labour care: relief of pain. *British Medical Journal*, **318**, 927–30.

Kitzinger, S. (1997). *The New Pregnancy and Childbirth*. Penguin Books.

The National Childbirth Trust (2000). *The Complete Book of Pregnancy* (D. Metland, ed.), p. 89. The National Childbirth Trust and Thorsons.

Noble, E. (1995). *Essential Exercises for the Childbearing Year*, pp. 55–8. New Life Images.

Sleep, J. M. and Grant, A. (1987). Pelvic floor exercises in postnatal care. *Midwifery*, **3**, 158–64.

Sutton, J. (2000). Birth without active pushing and a physiological second stage of labour. *The Practising Midwife*, **3**(4), 32–4.

Chapter 13

Meeting the needs of fathers

This chapter discusses the needs and perspectives of fathers, and suggests ways of working with fathers so that they feel included, cared for, and prepared for the challenges of birth and parenthood. Although the focus is on men, many of the issues we discuss also apply to lesbian partners (see Chapter 17).

Men expecting babies

Although some women are single parents, many have a partner. Expectant fathers have real and legitimate needs. These should be addressed, not only because the well-being of fathers is essential for the well-being of the mother and baby, but also because the father too is facing one of the biggest life changes he is ever likely to experience. Everything is shifting; his relationship with his partner, his perceptions of himself, his lifestyle, and his relationships with his parents, her parents and with his peers. He may be concerned about restricted freedom, increased responsibility and his capacity to earn. He may be ambivalent about the pregnancy and becoming a father, as well as worried about his partner's well-being, the health of the baby and his own ability to offer support.

The rapid change in men's involvement in pregnancy, birth and early parenting means that most men lack positive male role models in these areas. The presence of men in antenatal classes and in the labour ward is relatively recent, and only became standard practice during the last quarter of the twentieth century. Before that, a man who wanted to be present at a hospital birth, who carried his baby in a sling or pushed a buggy was thought to be odd. Now, a man who is not actively involved is often regarded negatively. Almost within one generation, assumptions about men's roles moved from one extreme to the other, with little leeway for individual reflection and choice.

Men's own fathers may not have been actively involved in their birth and care as infants. Some have lost touch with their fathers as result of family breakdown. They may not have any contact with men of their own age who are already fathers. Media images do not help, as positive role models are few and far between. Portrayals of fathers are often mocking, their concerns tend to be ridiculed, and they are they often depicted as absent, unsupportive, inadequate or abusive (Burgess, 1997, pp. 19–20, 23). It is not surprising therefore that some men feel uncertain about their new role.

At the same time, gender conditioning can affect men's ability to acknowledge their concerns and their willingness to seek support. Male conditioning affects different men differently. However, like women, men are strongly influenced by the expectations that society and their peers have of them. The stereotypical man is tough, strong, decisive, knowledgeable, competitive and in control. He may equate masculinity with dominance, and resort to aggression when he feels threatened or powerless. He downplays and disguises any feelings of helplessness, uncertainty, weakness or sensitivity, does not admit to anxiety or fear, and does not cry (Clare, 2000).

Of course the male stereotype is a generalization – personalities and attitudes vary from person to person. In addition, society's expectations of men are constantly changing, and many men adapt accordingly. Most men want to be supportive because they love their partner and want them and the baby to be safe. However, many men are likely to be confused and uncertain about their role (Lewis, 1999). They are more likely than women to be isolated, and less likely to talk about relationships, feelings and fears. Some may have children by previous partners. One or two, perhaps unbeknown to their current partners, may be reminded of babies they fathered that were aborted.

Yet a great deal is expected of a man during pregnancy and labour and as a father. Society tacitly demands a complete role reversal. A man is suddenly required to be gentle, sensitive, intuitive and aware, qualities that in other settings might be labelled unmanly. In the labour ward he is expected to be a 'hand maiden', and to cope, with little or no preparation or support, with unpredictability, powerlessness and the stress of seeing his partner in pain and difficulty without being unable to do much about it (Hallgren *et al.*, 1999). Men may feel better if they can provide practical help in labour, but women may prefer 'quiet support', which can be harder to give (Somers-Smith, 1999).

Despite these demands, men often receive little input and support. They are seldom encouraged to express their needs and feelings, and may not be offered the support, skills and information they need. In short, the father is 'the most neglected member of the family' (Bennett, 1998).

Good antenatal classes can offer men a unique opportunity to prepare for birth and fatherhood. However, classes do not always meet fathers' needs (Nolan, 1994; Donovan, 1995; Smith, 1999a), and some classes are 'endured and not enjoyed' (Barclay *et al.*, 1996). Some men are keen to come to support their partners and to learn alongside them (Smith, 1999a). However, many do not know what to expect, and some may be genuinely worried about what might be expected of them. As one father said to us, 'it was like entering a women's Masonic lodge'. Smith (1999b) describes three attitudes to classes amongst the fathers in her study – 'totally committed, passive accepter or reluctant attender'. Satisfyingly, she found that when class content and structure were relevant to men's needs, reluctant attenders became committed.

Starting with yourself

Your attitudes towards fathers will have a profound influence on your classes, and will affect their tone far more than your teaching techniques or the exercises you use. If you are able to choose whether you will include fathers, your attitudes towards them may lead you to decide for or against couples' classes, or influence the number of sessions to which you invite fathers.

For some class leaders, having men in the class is problematic. Some are not sure why men are there; others say that the presence of men inhibits women from talking freely, or that men will distract the group with too many jokes or even outright hostility. Some leaders believe that childbearing is essentially women's business, and that the focus should be on their needs and feelings. Others are concerned about alienating women who are without a partner. Others, when pressed, admit that they feel anxious about leading mixed sex groups, perhaps because they find it hard to believe that men will take them seriously.

However, other class leaders counter these negative views with more positive ones. They say that any disadvantages can be minimized and managed, that men widen the scope of classes, and that having them there simply reflects the reality of two-parent families. Helping men will also, in turn, benefit women and their babies. Classes that include men's needs allow the women to relax and pay attention to their own needs rather than endlessly worrying whether their partners are bored, angry or alienated. And having both men and women in a group greatly increases the overall richness and variety and helps the group work well.

Take a moment to reflect on your attitudes and assumptions. How do you feel about having fathers in your classes? If you are female, your views are likely to be influenced by your own experiences in relation to men, for example as daughter, sister, niece, girlfriend, partner, mother of sons and so on. Are you influenced by media images of men and childbirth, or by stereotypical views expressed by colleagues? Have you had difficulties with men in your classes? Do you believe that birth should be women's business? Or is it a question of your self-confidence?

Finding out what men think and need

Like the women they accompany, men bring with them their own feelings and needs as well as a lifetime of experience. Class leaders are much more likely to be aware of the practical and emotional needs of pregnant women than of expectant fathers. If that's true of you, take any opportunity you can to invite men to talk, and then listen really well.

The key to doing this is to listen to men when their partners are not there. This is crucial if you want to hear what men really think and feel. When women are present, *their* perspective tends to creep in and then take over. If you have listened to couples talking about the birth, you will almost certainly have heard a woman say to her partner, 'No, it wasn't like that at all. You've got it all wrong'. Men tend to censor what they say in order to protect their partner. Although many men are frightened that their partner could die in labour, they will not mention the possibility whilst sitting next to her. Some men keep quiet about their own concerns because they do not want to seem selfish (Szeverényi *et al.*, 1998; Somers-Smith, 1999).

So take every opportunity to listen to men. You could divide your class into single sex groups (see below), or invite only the men from a class back to talk together after their babies have been born. Listen to male friends, relatives or colleagues. Listen to fathers whenever you can – after the birth, during home visits. Even a brief 'How are you?' at the door or while the mother is busy elsewhere can be supportive to the father and enlightening for you. One new father burst into tears when asked this question, and said, 'Nobody else has asked me that. Not even my own mother'.

There are a whole range of questions you could ask to give you the insights you need to work well with expectant fathers. For example:

- how did you feel during your partner's pregnancy? What changes did you notice in yourself? Who or what helped?
- what it was like for you coming to classes? What was good? What was hard? What else would have been useful?
- what was it like for you being at the labour and at your baby's birth? What did you feel prepared for? What would you have liked to have known more about?
- what was it like leaving your partner and your baby in hospital after the birth? How did you get home? How did you feel?
- what was it like bringing your partner and baby home? What did you feel prepared for? What would you have liked to have known more about?
- so far, what has been good and what has been hard about life with a new baby? What did you feel prepared for? What would you have liked to have known more about?
- what else do you think we should be saying to fathers in antenatal classes?

In time, you will hear a wide range of experiences and begin to recognize common issues and reactions. Listening to men on a regular basis will help you gauge whether or not your classes are meeting their needs. It will also enable you to be a conduit between new fathers and expectant fathers. A useful phrase is 'What many fathers say is ...'. Hearing what other men have said may be, for many men, a more acceptable way of taking on new ideas than being told what to expect by a health professional, especially if she is a woman. You have only to reverse the process and imagine how some women are likely to react if a man tells them how they will feel and what they should do.

Welcoming and involving fathers

Men can't just be tacked on to a women's course. They have to be included all along the way, from planning and publicity, to the actual work you do together.

Include a specific welcome to fathers in all written and verbal invitations to couples' classes and to fathers' evenings.

Consider every topic and activity from the father's point of view. Traditionally, classes, books and written material have focused mainly on the women's perspectives (Singh and Newburn, 2000) and perhaps on ways in which fathers can offer support. Men who come to classes are usually keen to know what they can do to help, but helping strategies alone are unlikely to prepare them for what they will experience. If you have tried the *Labour Line* (see Chapter 9), you will have a graphic visual image of the length of labour and of very limited amount the father can actually *do*. There are likely to be long periods when all he can do is just 'be there'. This is the hardest role of all for many people, regardless of gender.

Include the father's perspective not only as a supporter, but also as a human being who is experiencing life-changing events. What will he see and hear? What might he smell or touch? What feelings might the experience trigger in him? What information will he need to make sense of what is happening? What can he do to take care of his own needs and feelings? Try doing this for every single topic and issue that might arise during an antenatal course. Consider what you would say to a men-only group. Would you change what you say when women are present?

If you have not had much opportunity to listen to men describing their experiences, you may find standing in a man's shoes surprisingly hard. If so, try thinking back to your student days. How did you feel and react the first time you saw: a woman during a long and difficult labour; crowning; a forceps delivery; a woman with postnatal depression?

Having decided what to say to fathers, you need to develop ways of conveying different perspectives to the women and to the men in your class. For example, consider how you could talk to a mixed group about episiotomy. There are certain things that they both need to know, such as when, how and why it is done. Women might also need to know, for example, what the snip feels like, that a local anaesthetic sometimes stings, that looking with a mirror afterwards helps give a true picture of the scar size, and ways to speed healing.

Men, on the other hand, need to know what they can expect to witness. For example, the snip itself is audible and some men say it is upsetting to watch it being done. They need to be offered ways of coping – hum quietly when the midwife picks up the scissors; instead of watching, be at the head of the bed to support your partner. They may welcome suggestions on more comfortable lovemaking afterwards. Or you might suggest ways to help a woman as she is being stitched. When you cover a topic in this way, some of the class is 'eavesdropping' so you will need to switch from one to the other frequently, clearly signalling whom you are addressing (see Chapter 6).

As well as topics common to both men and women, think about the things that only fathers may experience – what you could say that would prepare them for what they might do, and also how other men have said they felt and what helped them. For example, topics may include:

- arranging to leave work at a moment's notice when labour starts
- being a labour supporter and the feelings that this can evoke
- taking care of himself
- seeing his partner in pain or difficulty
- witnessing the birth of their baby
- being left abruptly outside the theatre during an emergency Caesarean birth
- being separated from his partner and baby when he leaves the hospital
- juggling the demands of a job, visiting hospital, keeping the home in some semblance of order and fielding calls from relatives
- negotiating paternity leave or days off work to be with his partner and baby when they come home from hospital
- having to go to work despite sleepless nights
- managing the conflicting demands of work and family life.

One issue that is often not tackled in classes is whether men want to be present at the birth. Although many men say that they would not have missed it for the world, and both men and women can benefit from being there together, it is important not to assume that his being there is the best thing for everyone. Some men may be terrified and squeamish. For some men, witnessing the birth has a profoundly negative effect on their emotional and sexual relationships with their partners (O'Driscoll, 1994). Class leaders can help couples to decide what is best for them by giving clear information about the physical and emotional realities of being a labour supporter, by offering the men practical suggestions about giving support and about caring for themselves, and by giving them space to reflect (Bartels, 1999).

Another neglected topic is what men do after the birth, especially at night. Most men will have missed at least one and possibly two or even three nights sleep. They will not have eaten properly for many hours, and will have been through an extremely demanding and emotional experience. In the absence of rooming-in facilities, fathers are often encouraged to 'go home and sleep'. So they need to think about how they will get home and what support they might need. Public transport may not be available. Driving is not the safest option. We have heard from several midwives in different parts of the UK of sleep-deprived fathers having accidents on the way home and, tragically, of one fatality. Some fathers may welcome the opportunity to return to the peace and quiet of home, but others find it hard to be alone after such a momentous experience. Antenatal classes can offer fathers time to reflect on various options – for example, having cash for a taxi, calling a friend to pick them up, staying with family or friends and so on – and decide what they would prefer to do.

Involve fathers in everything

This means making sure that your language is always inclusive (see Chapter 6). You may also need to consider the generic term you use for the people in the room who are not pregnant. Most leaders have long abandoned 'husbands', but what word(s) will replace it? Partners? Dads? Fathers? Men? You guys? How will you address a group if it includes a lesbian couple or a woman and her female friend or mother? All these variations will demand a change in the words you use.

Always involve men in practical work. Some may be very reluctant to join in, but with gentle encouragement most can be persuaded that this will be less awkward than sitting on the sidelines as a spectator. Invite them to try out relaxation and breathing for themselves. Offer time for men to receive massage before they give it. Encourage them to help their partners find comfortable positions, and to explore ways of supporting their partners both physically and emotionally.

During these activities, make sure that men look after themselves. Watch posture and positioning so that they avoid straining their backs when they support or massage their partners. Acknowledge how tiring it can be helping a woman in labour. Look at ways to ease the harder bits, and identify the things that men can do to conserve their energy. These will include wearing cool clothing, eating regularly, and taking time for a stretch and perhaps a breath of fresh air.

Fathers are expected to take an active part in caring for their babies, and therefore have the same needs for information and skills as new mothers. Couples who learn together start off on an equal basis, while fathers who are left to learn from their partners can be at a disadvantage (Burgess, 1997, pp. 131–5). Whether you are working with groups or individuals, antenatally and postnatally, involve men whenever you discuss or demonstrate practical aspects of infant care.

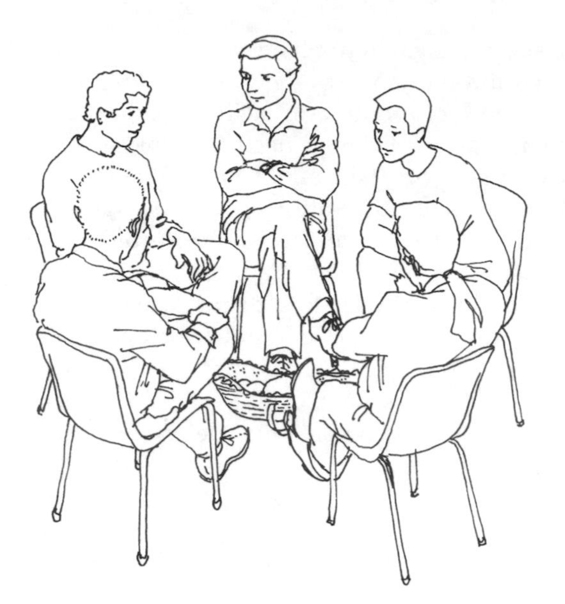

Figure 13.1

Create opportunities for peer support

Antenatal classes can offer men a unique opportunity to talk with other men in the same situation. This is more likely to happen in single sex groups. You can either hold a fathers' only evening or, when the group is well established, divide the class into single-sex groups (Figure 13.1). If you have a mixture of male and female partners, you will need to work out whether it is appropriate for male and female supporters to be together, or whether they need separate groups. The best way to decide is to ask the participants what they would prefer.

If you want men to talk really freely, you will need to set some groundrules about feedback before you start. Feedback is not really necessary. Sometimes, simply giving people time and safety in which to talk and listen is enough. Not reporting back to the whole class often spurs couples into talking together after the class. If this is the plan, say so when you set up the groups, and remind people that anything that is said in their group must remain confidential or be shared in a way that respects others' anonymity. If you want sub-groups to report back, they need to know both if and how it is to be done before they begin. One way to do this that preserves confidentiality is to ask groups to summarize their discussions on a chart. The charts can then be displayed and discussed in a way that maintains confidentiality for individuals. This often triggers an interesting exchange about different and similar perspectives. Here are some suggested questions to trigger discussions in single sex groups.

- 'How do you feel about the prospect of labour?'

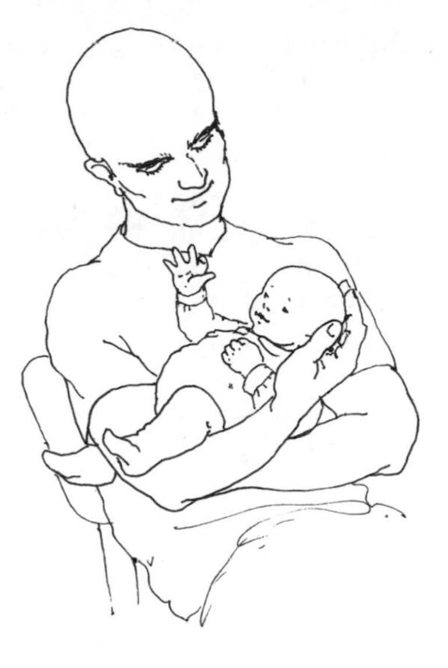

Figure 13.2

- 'What do you think will be good about being a father/mother? What will be hard?

Offer positive and practical images of fatherhood

Because men have few models and few positive images of fatherhood, you can help them by offering realistic and practical insights. One way of doing this is to start a discussion on what men have heard from their male friends and relatives about being at the birth and becoming a father.

Check your visual aids, especially slides and videos, for inclusiveness. Many marginalize the father, focusing instead on the woman and midwife. Anything you show to a mixed group should depict an involved and active man rather than an anxious-looking one sitting awkwardly in the corner. You could balance the focus on mothers by displaying a collage of fathers holding, changing, soothing, bathing or playing with their babies.

Another way is to invite a new father to talk about his experience of labour, birth and the early days of parenting (see Chapter 15).

Key points

- The class leader's attitudes to men have a profound effect on their ability to meet fathers' needs.
- Men expecting babies are facing a major life change. A great deal is expected of them, but often they do not receive the support that they need.

- Men may be reluctant to voice their own needs and concerns, especially when their partner is present.
- Men's needs should be considered, from planning and publicity to the actual content and style of the antenatal course.
- It is important to:
  - consider every topic from the father's viewpoint, both as supporter and as a person with his own needs and feelings
  - include topics that are specific to fathers
  - involve fathers in every activity and use inclusive language
  - create opportunities for peer support
  - offer positive images of fatherhood.

References

Barclay, L., Donovan, J. and Genovese, A.(1996). Men's experiences during their partner's first pregnancy: a grounded theory analysis. *Australian Journal of Advanced Nursing*, **13**(3), 12–24.

Bartels, R. (1999). Experience of childbirth from the father's perspective. *British Journal of Midwifery*, **7**(11), 861–3.

Bennett, H. J. (1998). Apgar scores for dads. *British Medical Journal*, **317**, 1712.

Burgess, A. (1997). *Fatherhood Reclaimed: The Making of the Modern Father*. Vermilion, an imprint of Ebury Press.

Clare, A. (2000). *On Men: Masculinity in Crisis*. Chatto and Windus.

Donovan, J. (1995). The process of analysis during a grounded theory study of men during their partners' pregnancies. *Journal of Advanced Nursing*, **21**, 708–15.

Hallgren, A., Kihlgren, M. and Forslin, L. (1999). Swedish fathers' involvement in experiences of childbirth preparation and childbirth. *Midwifery*, **15**, 6–15.

Lewis, C. (1999). Transition to fatherhood. In: *Transition to Parenting: An Open Learning Resource for Midwives*. The Royal College of Midwives Trust.

Nolan, M. (1994). Caring for fathers in antenatal classes. *Modern Midwife*, **4**(2), 25–8.

O'Driscoll, M. (1994). Midwives, childbirth and sexuality. 2: Men and sex. *British Journal of Midwifery*, **2**(2), 74–6.

Singh, D. and Newburn, M. (2000). *Becoming a Father: Men's Access to Information and Support about Pregnancy, Birth and Life with a New Baby*. The National Childbirth Trust.

Smith, N. (1999a). Antenatal classes and the transition to fatherhood: a study of some fathers' views. *MIDIRS Midwifery Digest*, **9**(4), 463–8.

Smith, N. (1999b). Antenatal classes and the transition to fatherhood: a study of some fathers' views. *MIDIRS Midwifery Digest*, **9**(3), 327–30.

Somers-Smith, M. J. (1999). A place for the partner? Expectations and experience of support during childbirth. *Midwifery*, **15**, 101–8.
Szeverényi, P., Póka, R., Hetey M. and Török, Z. (1998). Contents of birth-related fear among couples wishing the partner's presence at delivery. *Journal of Psychosomatic Obstetrics and Gynaecology*, **19**(1), 38–43.

Chapter 14

Sensitive topics

This chapter suggests ways of dealing with topics that may make you uneasy. If the issues we discuss don't match your own particular worries, concentrate on the approach. We cannot promise that reading this chapter will make everything easy. However, with some planning and practice, you can talk as fluently about sensitive issues as you can about any other topic.

Starting with yourself

How do you handle sensitive topics at the moment? A few leaders avoid some or all of them altogether, either because the topic is hard to handle or because there seems little point in worrying expectant parents about things that might never happen. Others say they are willing to cover anything, as long as it is brought up by someone in the class. Some ensure that certain topics are always included unless a situation arises in a particular class that leads them to adapt their usual practice. Are there topics that you find difficult to handle? Do you include the following topics in your course?

	Always	Never	Sometimes
Birth options (e.g. home birth)			
Mobility throughout labour			
Pain in labour			
The disadvantages and side effects of:			
• technology and interventions			
• drugs			
Sex during pregnancy			
Sex after birth			
Stillbirth			
Neonatal intensive care			

	Always	Never	Sometimes
Cot death			
Postnatal depression			
Exhaustion after birth			

What makes it difficult?

When we ask class leaders what makes them dread or avoid certain topics, they list concerns about raising anxiety, upsetting people, 'opening cans of worms', and not having the time or the confidence to deal with what might come up. With some topics, the problem is their own embarrassment and their fear of embarrassing parents. A few may be concerned about what is and is not appropriate to discuss with people of minority cultures and religions (see Chapter 17).

Raising anxiety

Many people assume that stress and anxiety are always negative and should be avoided, yet without them we would lack motivation, be unable to develop coping strategies, and remain unprepared for challenging and stressful situations. 'There seems to be an optimum amount of fear for good performance' (Marks, 1978).

Some anxiety is inevitable during pregnancy. In fact, the absence of anxiety would be surprising in the face of the enormous physical, emotional, social and practical challenges of pregnancy, and the prospect of birth and parenthood:

> *All women worry about childbirth, so the frank antenatal teacher is not going to create anxieties which do not exist already. S/he may however temporarily suppress them and create a reassuring vision of childbirth which is unlikely to be fulfilled*
>
> (Niven, 1992, p. 60)

Although high levels of anxiety and distress during pregnancy can be damaging (Niven, 1992, p. 33), a certain amount of anxiety can actually help women prepare for the realities of labour, especially if it encourages them to develop coping strategies – 'Anticipatory distress can have advantages provided it leads to problem-solving behaviour' (Craig, 1999). Attempts to suppress anxiety may work in the short term, but reassurance that creates unrealistic expectations leaves people unprepared for the actual experience. As a result, they may end up feeling let down and angry, and may blame themselves for failing to have the kind of birth they anticipated (Niven, 1992, p. 61).

Although sharing fears and discussing the realities of labour can raise anxiety in the short term, there are also overall benefits. Sharing fears and knowing 'it's not just you' can in itself be helpful. Some fears may be unfounded and can be allayed – 'We don't do shaves and enemas any more'. Others can be put into perspective – 'There have been rare cases of paralysis after an epidural, but statistically, crossing the road is much more risky'. Parents can also learn coping strategies –'Yes, contractions can get extremely painful, let's go through some of the things that can help'.

Embarrassment

The discomfort of embarrassment is very unpleasant. However, ignoring potentially embarrassing topics can mean that people do not have information that could prevent or alleviate problems. As a class leader or health professional, you will already be accustomed to discussing topics that you are unlikely to talk about in other circumstances. With some planning and practice, we can all learn to deal with topics that can be embarrassing.

Opening cans of worms

Some leaders avoid or skim over certain topics, fearing that if they say too much or encourage people to think too deeply they could make matters worse rather than better. Classes cannot and should not be psychotherapeutic encounter groups, but they can offer opportunities for parents to reflect. For example, a woman who has not thought about the effect of a new baby on family and social relationships may end up overwhelmed by visitors and advice, or be isolated and struggling to cope. The needs and feelings of men who are ambivalent about being present at the birth may be ignored, glossed over or trivialized (see Chapter 13). Questions such as 'What will you do that your parents did? What will you do differently?' might indeed raise sensitive issues and strong feelings, but raising them also makes it possible for people to make conscious and thoughtful choices and plans.

Dealing with what might come up

In any group there is always a chance that someone might hint at or talk about potentially distressing issues and difficulties. Although this can create short-term discomfort for everyone present, it does offer the person a chance to let off steam and to reflect, which can bring long-term benefits. It also enables others to offer support and suggest sources of help (see 'Managing strong feelings' in Chapter 7).

Not enough time

Many of us assume that all this is bound to be messy and take up too much time, but this is not necessarily so. People rarely get a chance to talk without interruption while others just listen with respect. Blau (1989) observed that, given time to talk without interruption, few of his patients talked longer than two or three minutes. You can help enormously by allowing the person a bit of class time and offering more time later. You can also refer people to other sources of help and support.

Short-term pain for long-term gain

If leaders allow their own fears to dominate their decisions about what to include in classes, parents may lose out. Leaders need to consider and meet parents' longer-term needs. Although discussing difficult and painful subjects can be hard, parents are more likely to be realistic and better prepared. They are less likely to say afterwards, 'I had no idea how painful and long labour could be', or 'I didn't realize how exhausting and tough the first few weeks were going to be', or 'I didn't know that epidurals could lead to so much intervention'. Here are some responses from class leaders who were asked to list the immediate and long-term benefits and disadvantages of raising sensitive topics:

- Short- and long-term *advantages* to parents include: being more prepared; increased confidence; better coping strategies; able to be more flexible and adaptable; unnecessary fear can be allayed; the fantasy is sometimes worse than reality; able to function better if realistic; personal growth; likely to feel more positive after the event.
- Short- and long-term *disadvantages* to parents include: raised anxiety; reduced confidence; creating self-fulfilling prophecies.

Try this analysis for yourself. Take a topic you find difficult. Decide on the three things you could say that parents have a right to know about, and that might benefit them in the long term. Would including the topic, even briefly, be more honest and realistic than omitting it? Then list the short- and long-term disadvantages of including it. It is easy to allow our own anxieties to influence what we list and do not list, so ask colleagues and friends to add their ideas.

If the long-term advantages outweigh the disadvantages, perhaps you should include the topic. It is worth remembering that, even if you decide to exclude certain topics, sooner or later they will be raised by a participant. Giving some thought to how you will respond when this happens is time well spent.

How much should we say?

Too little information can result in parents feeling unprepared, patronized, confused or angry. They cannot make informed choices, and are less likely to cope with the challenges of birth and early parenthood – in short, they are disempowered. Too much information is equally disempowering as it can raise unnecessary anxiety and confusion. The really essential information is more likely to be forgotten, and parents may feel overwhelmed by the amount that they have heard.

Finding the balance between too little and too much information for a group of people is not easy. 'Vigilant' people want to know everything, and 'deniers' prefer to know very little. Interestingly, there is evidence that 'deniers' simply do not take in what they do not want to hear (Niven, 1992, pp. 61–63). Most people are between these two extremes, and we have found the best way to get the level of information about right for the majority of people is to use the following method:

- Stick to the principle of telling them three essential things. If the topic is sensitive, you will need to choose your 'three things' with care, finding a balance between glossing over the issue and making it sound unbearably awful.
- Include information about how women and their partners might *feel*, so that they are prepared for the actual experience (Niven, 1992, p. 65).
- Whenever possible, balance what you say with a positive aspect – 'Contractions can be very painful, but they come and go so you can rest in between them'; 'Each contraction brings the birth of your baby one step closer'.
- Offer coping strategies. What can parents do themselves that can help? What other help is available? It is interesting to note that although cot death is a topic that people shy away from, health professionals tell us that when infant resuscitation training is offered to parents, attendance levels are usually high.
- Then, form small groups of not more than four people and suggest that they discuss what they think and what they would like to know more about.
- Next, invite comments and questions from the whole group. This gives you a chance to find out what else people need. Pay attention to people's reactions, and listen attentively to what people say. Make sure that you respond to everyone who wants to talk. If one person asks for much more information than the rest, you could offer individual attention outside class time (see Chapter 19).
- End by acknowledging that the topic has been difficult, and move on to something positive and enjoyable (for example, see 'Advert for parents of a newborn baby' in Chapter 9). Avoid coffee breaks and relaxation sessions immediately after dealing with a sensitive topic, as these can leave individuals isolated.

Below we discuss a few topics that many people find difficult.

Talking about sex

Many of us find it hard to talk openly about sex. We may be unsure of our ground, or afraid that others will be embarrassed or offended. This reticence is not surprising. Although there is an appearance of sexual liberation in our society, sex is still surrounded by secrecy and taboos. But if you shy away, is it for your benefit or for theirs? Pregnancy and the arrival of a new baby have such an enormous impact on a couple's whole relationship, and on their sexual relationship in particular. You will do them a service by raising the issues and making information available in your class.

What do parents want to know?

Most people have questions about sex that they would like to ask, but don't. Many find it reassuring to know, that barring obstetric problems, sexual intercourse is safe throughout pregnancy, neither damaging the baby nor triggering a labour that is not already imminent. It is also helpful to know that some people want to be more sexually active during pregnancy, while others lose interest – sometimes completely. This can be true of both men and women, and can cause major stress if partners are out of step with each other. The group may be reassured to know that this is common, and that talking things through and understanding each other's feelings can help.

Sexual problems after birth are very common. Parents may find it helpful to know that after a birth, many women are uninterested in any sexual activity. Penetrative sex in particular can be problematic, perhaps because of exhaustion, soreness after stitching, or the slow return of natural vaginal secretions. Some new mothers feel too involved with the baby to make space for their partner's needs.

New fathers describe changes too. Some are put off by what happened at the birth, or by changes in their partner's body. Many are afraid of causing pain. Most couples say that it takes time, gentleness and understanding to resume any kind of active sex life. It is often years before anything like pre-baby sex returns (Barrett *et al.*, 2000; Bartellas *et al.*, 2000).

If your class doesn't provide this information, where else will they hear it? There is evidence that many people have very little information, and that few people approach health professionals for help (Barrett *et al.*, 2000). Being informed can help parents to avoid or minimize problems and anxieties. We find this a persuasive argument for including discussion about sex in antenatal classes. Take some time to think about what information you will offer to help parents cope with the effect of pregnancy, birth and parenthood on their sex life.

How to discuss sex

Once you have decided what to say, think through the vocabulary you will use with the group (see also Chapters 6 and 17). Practise what you want to say by talking out loud or using a tape recorder. You may not want to go as far as the class leader who sat in front of a mirror saying 'penis' over and over again until it felt alright – but what *can* you do to reduce embarrassment and awkwardness? The more confident and relaxed you are in your approach, the more receptive and open your class members will be.

When to raise the topic

Sex in pregnancy should be discussed as soon as possible, and not left until just before the women are about to give birth. However, the idea of sex after birth won't seem relevant early in the course. There are lots of ways to introduce the subject. For example, when teaching pelvic floor exercises right at the beginning of the course, you could mention practising during sexual intercourse. If the class discusses changes in pregnancy, you could say, 'What about sex? Any differences?'. Towards the end of the course you may spend time on the changes parenthood brings, or lead a discussion on contraception. It may appear in the 'safe pot' (see Chapter 5), or you could put it in yourself.

Another way to give information is to display books and leaflets that deal with sex during pregnancy and after the birth. Participants can acquire the information they need or augment the information you have given. However, written material does not appeal to everyone. Those who are not used to learning through reading will have to rely on you.

Talking about stillbirth

Since stillbirth is relatively rare, there may seem little purpose in raising the issue, especially as many class leaders worry that they are creating anxiety where it doesn't already exist. In reality, almost all expectant parents have either thought or dreamt about this possibility, although few voice their fears. While it is true that they become subdued when stillbirth is mentioned, people later say it was helpful that the unmentionable was given a voice. It is the only topic we have ever been thanked for including in the course!

What information might be helpful?

Apart from acknowledging the reality of stillbirth, there are certain pieces of information parents say are helpful. Notice that the statements below – unlike most of what you say to the group – are deliberately *not* directed at the listening parents.

- Most stillborn babies look normal, and seeing and holding the baby can be very helpful. The reality of the baby's appearance is almost always better than the fantasy, and having time to meet and then say goodbye to their baby helps parents in the long term (SANDS, 1995).

- It's routine in many places for the staff to do things that can help parents to remember their baby. For example, they may take photographs, locks of hair, foot- and handprints.
- Naming the baby and perhaps arranging a funeral can also help parents acknowledge and grieve their loss.
- Support networks are available for both parents. Fathers grieve too, and need as much support as mothers.

Parents can only hold a few thoughts because they are so distracted by their emotions. Pare down what you say to the absolute essentials. Remember that for some people some of the routines after a stillbirth may be unacceptable on cultural and religious grounds (Schott and Henley, 1996). Hearing in advance what is usually offered may help people to clarify what is or is not acceptable to them.

How and when to discuss stillbirth

There are several ways in which the subject of stillbirth can be raised, either by developing your own openings or by staying alert for any the group offers. These include:

- in response to newspaper radio and television stories
- in a 'safe pot' exercise (see Chapter 5)
- any time dreams are mentioned. Many pregnant women (and some partners) have very vivid dreams – perhaps that the baby is dead, or born able to walk and talk. You can comment that it is common for people to dream that, for example, something is wrong with the baby, and that many parents have that fear buried somewhere. It's also worth mentioning that thinking or dreaming about stillbirth or abnormality does not signify that anything is wrong, or cause it to happen!

However well you time the introduction and however sensitively you handle what happens next, discussing stillbirth is depressing and the atmosphere in the class always becomes quiet and heavy. It's important to acknowledge this, and then to ensure that there is plenty of time to lighten the mood and regain a sense of proportion before the class ends. Here are some points to keep in mind:

- If you bring it up, do so in the first half of a class and in the first two-thirds of the course.
- If someone else brings it up and you cannot handle it well, perhaps because you lack the time to do so, acknowledge the speaker, offer individual time, and deal with the immediate needs of the group. If it is appropriate, spend some time on the topic in the next class.
- Follow the discussion with time to let off steam in small groups, then change the mood by doing something lively and practical. You may

want to ask the following week if there are any repercussions following what was said at the previous session.

When a baby dies

If someone in your class has a baby who dies, you yourself will need support. You will also need to decide what support you will offer the bereaved parents. Finally, there is the decision as to whether and how the rest of the group will be told.

Parents whose babies are stillborn or die soon after birth are bound to feel that they have failed. They may associate you only with positive outcomes and healthy babies, and feel that they are no longer entitled to your attention. However, your acknowledgement of their status as parents who have suffered a real loss can be very helpful, whereas withdrawal is likely to accentuate their feelings of failure. You will need to work out what you can offer, and ensure that you get time to deal with your feelings both before and after you offer your support (see Chapter 21).

You will then need to think through how to approach the rest of the class. If you teach open classes it may not be obvious that someone is missing; however, if you teach a closed class or hold a reunion, the absence of class members is bound to be noticed. Will you wait until somebody asks, or will you break the news to them yourself? Some leaders think it is better not to tell the rest of the class unless someone asks, especially if they have not yet had their babies. They argue that it will only raise anxiety and distress. Others feel the opposite, finding it is easier for everyone if the leader decides when and how to break the news, since someone is bound to ask or find out sooner or later.

One compelling reason for telling the class is the benefit bereaved parents can feel when their group offers sympathy and support. Again and again, parents whose baby has died say that people avoid them, do not acknowledge their loss, and treat them as though they have never been parents (Kohner and Henley, 2001). By raising the matter publicly, you add to the whole community's ability to handle tragedy more sensitively.

Whatever course of action you decide on, it is important to discuss it first with the bereaved parents. They will have views, and their feelings and right to confidentiality must be respected.

If, with the parents' agreement, you tell the class, it is better to do it first thing and to break the news as simply as possible. The amount of detail you give will depend on the bereaved parents' wishes. Allow time for people to assimilate the news and perhaps talk about how they feel in small groups of not more than three women or two couples. One way that can help the group to express sympathy is to send a joint card, signed by everyone in the class.

Some groups will need a long time to mull things over, while others will want to move on more quickly. You will need to judge how long to give them. Follow on by putting this sad event into proportion. Help the group to see that stillbirth is uncommon and the chances of it happening are small – perhaps link it to everyday risks like driving a car, which accounts for more deaths than stillbirth. Afterwards, choose an activity that will lighten the atmosphere, although it is probably unrealistic to expect to send everyone home feeling happy.

This will have been a hard class to lead, so afterwards get some support for yourself before you go on to your next task. If you can arrange this in advance, so much the better.

Talking about birth options, technology and intervention

Class leaders vary considerably in their approach to discussing birth options, medical interventions and obstetric technology. It's not just class leaders who have polarized views; parents have them, too. The people who come to your class will hold a whole cross-section of attitudes about how babies should be born, the role of technology in pregnancy and labour, and how involved they want to be in the decision-making process. Some expect health professionals to make decisions for them and are surprised that others want to be involved when there are 'experts' to do it for them. A few are determined to maintain control of what happens to them at all costs, and are suspicious of (or downright hostile towards) any advice they are offered. A common middle way is to be interested in a handful of choices, concentrating on getting them 'right', and taking a more passive approach to the rest.

The job of the class leader is to help everyone to be flexible and open-minded. That's the best way to enable people to make good decisions. Seeing only one side of any issue is liable to leave people disappointed or disillusioned, and occasionally it leads to battles between carers and parents. Very rarely, when diametrically opposed views have led to a breakdown in two-way communication, people may take unnecessary risks or may land up with avoidable confrontation.

Class leaders need to set aside any strong views and offer full, balanced and accurate information about what is involved, the advantages and disadvantages, and the indications and contraindications. This isn't easy. If you work in a hospital setting where choice is limited by standardized care and the use of technology is routine, you may feel it is unwise to discuss the drawbacks of routine monitoring, artificial rupture of the membranes, epidurals or Caesarean sections. The argument goes, 'If that's what is in store for parents, why make it harder for them?'.

On the other hand, you may believe so strongly in natural birth and be so aware of the disadvantages of technology and obstetric management that you find it hard to give appropriate time to discussing them at all, let alone their benefits. Or you might be so accustomed to high-tech birth that you simply can't see why anyone would want a physiological alternative – 'Would you have your appendix out without anaesthesia?'.

Actually, these views are more like caricatures than reality. Most of us fall somewhere between these extremes. Where do you fit in? Can you be as open-minded as you would like parents to be? Unless you can, you will not offer parents the assistance they deserve to help them face what may be difficult choices.

Taking the middle road is not the same as sitting on the fence. It means knowing your hobbyhorses and deciding not to ride them. It means paying close attention to what you say and how you say it. It means offering parents ways of making the best decisions they can given their own circumstances, beliefs and experience; and then accepting that their views may not in any way resemble yours. It can't be done without regular reviews of current evidence and regular assessments of your own beliefs and attitudes.

Talking about pain

Most women describe labour pain as severe or very severe (Melzack, 1984), yet the nature and potential intensity of the sensations and the pain that typically occur in labour are often not fully addressed in antenatal classes. Underplaying pain may be seen as protective, but it can be counterproductive. When expectations do not match reality, women can experience unnecessary and sometimes devastating levels of fear and anxiety. This can have lasting effects on their relationship with health professionals and on their self-esteem (Niven, 1992, p. 61).

Parents need honest information about labour pain. They need to know that the severity and location of labour pain varies from woman to woman; and what the woman might experience at different stages – for example, the intense and often disturbing sensations of pressure on the rectum as the baby's head descends, and the feelings of stretching, burning and splitting as the baby's head stretches the perineum. The pain or discomfort women might experience postnatally could also be addressed – for example, what after-pains and a bruised or stitched perineum can feel like.

This realism must be combined with coping strategies (see Chapters 11 and 12). Psychological approaches also help (Bonica and Chadwick, 1989). Women vary in what they find helpful, so it is better to offer a range of ideas so that they can pick and choose images that appeal to them. For example, when talking about labour you could:

- start by inviting people to discuss their past experience of pain, what helped and what did not

- talk about 'pain with a purpose' or 'positive pain', or compare it to the pain experienced by marathon runners. This reduces fear by helping people to understand that, unlike all other pain, the pain of labour does not signal damage or harm, but in most cases is completely normal
- explain that for most women the pain stops between contractions, so they can rest in between
- suggest they treat every contraction as a separate entity. Some people might find it useful to imagine that, at the start of labour, there is a pile of contractions in their in-tray. As soon as a contraction is over it goes in the out-tray, so the pile to be dealt with decreases as the labour progresses
- encourage parents to focus on the present and deal only with what is happening at the moment. Let the rest take care of itself. Imagining how much worse it might get only increases fear and therefore tension and pain
- offer positive images – each contraction brings your baby one step closer
- suggest distraction techniques – 'Imagine yourself in a place that you love'; 'listen to your favourite music'; 'Concentrate on a vase of flowers or a picture that you like'.

Assessing your personal views

We seldom have the support we need to offer hard truths to parents. However, if you find yourself repeatedly shying away from telling things as they really are, you are probably doing so for your own needs and not the parents'.

If you find it hard to talk calmly and objectively about any topic, find a sympathetic listener and think out loud about your own experience and feelings. We know people who have done this about home birth. Others have mulled over their relationships with doctors, breast- versus bottle-feeding, mobility in labour, and even seemingly trivial matters like dummies. We are not suggesting that you have to change your attitudes and beliefs. However, unless you are fully aware of them it is very difficult to set them aside and give parents a balanced view.

Although one person's straightforward choice is another's 'red rag to a bull', the pattern of introspective questioning remains largely the same. Ask yourself:

- what do parents have a right to know about this topic? What might be the long-term advantages and disadvantages of discussing it?
- what am I *not* saying? Why? What am I stressing? Why?
- what is the basis for the information I give – my own belief, a traditional practice, a review of the research literature, the word of a powerful figure in the field – or what?

You may find it helpful to list the pros and cons of the topic or issue. Check the relevant research data or find out about the approaches that other leaders use, then review your approach.

Key points

- Most class leaders find some topics difficult to handle.
- Class leaders need to be aware of their own beliefs and attitudes in order to set them aside and provide parents with balanced and realistic information.
- A certain amount of anxiety is inherent in pregnancy.
- Reassurance can lead to a gap between expectations and the actual experience.
- Realistic preparation is nearly always helpful in the long run.
- It is important to include information about how women and their partners might *feel* is as well as objective descriptions of what will happen and why.
- Realism must be combined with coping strategies.

References

Barrett, G., Pendry, E., Peacock, J. *et al.* (2000). Women's sexual health after childbirth. *British Journal of Obstetrics and Gynaecology*, **107**(2), 186–95.

Bartellas, E., Crane, J. M., Daley, M. *et al.* (2000). Sexuality and sexual activity in pregnancy. *British Journal of Obstetrics and Gynaecology*, **107**(8), 964–8.

Blau, J. N. (1989). Time to let the patient speak. *British Medical Journal*, **298**, 39.

Bonica, J. J. and Chadwick, H. S. (1989). Labour pain. In: *Textbook of Pain* (P. Wall and R. Melzack, eds), 2nd edn, p. 487. Churchill Livingstone.

Craig, K. D. (1999). Emotions and psychology. In: *Textbook of Pain* (P. Wall and R. Melzack, eds), 2nd edn, p. 336. Churchill Livingstone.

Kohner, N. and Henley, A. (2001). *When a Baby Dies*. Routledge.

Marks, I. M. (1978). *Living With Fear*, p. 9. McGraw-Hill Paperbacks.

Melzack, J. (1984). The myth of painless childbirth. The John Bonica lecture. Pain, **19**, 321.

Niven, C. A. (1992). *Psychological Care for Families: Before, During and After Birth*. Butterworth-Heinemann.

SANDS (1995). *Pregnancy. Loss and the Death of a Baby. Guidelines for Professionals*, revised edition. Stillbirth and Neonatal Death Society.

Schott, J. and Henley, A. (1996). *Culture, Religion and Childbearing in a Multi-Racial Society*. Butterworth-Heinemann, pp. 192–8.

Chapter 15

Preparing for life after birth

This chapter outlines ways in which you can help expectant parents to prepare for the realities of early parenthood.

Why cover life after birth?

Parenthood is one of the greatest and most challenging responsibilities that most people ever face. It is the only job that people are expected to do for 24 hours a day, seven days a week, 52 weeks year, for the best part of two decades. Expectations of and demands on parents are constantly shifting. Social and economic factors alter, health information and fashions in childcare change. Parents are usually expected to adapt and get on with it without help, support or appreciation. They tend not to be noticed until things go wrong, and then mothers, in particular, are usually blamed rather than supported.

A growing recognition of the importance of good parenting has led to the formation of statutory and voluntary organizations that offer support, information and skills training to parents. So what role can class leaders play in preparing people for this complex and ever-changing role? We believe that class leaders are in an ideal situation to lay the foundations for effective parenting. They see expectant parents on a regular basis over several weeks, and have time to build up trust and rapport. They can raise issues, offer information, teach skills and suggest strategies for managing new demands. They can encourage people to share their hopes and concerns and to build their own support networks.

Some class leaders feel that it is hard to get expectant parents to look beyond birth, and anyway there is so much to say about labour that there is little time for anything else. Labour, crucial though it is, seldom lasts longer than 24 hours, so although this view is understandable, it has several negative consequences. It can become a self-fulfilling prophecy and perpetuate the myth that the birth is the goal. It also encourages the idea that people only become parents once their baby is born, even though the mother's body is already nurturing and protecting the baby, and expectant parents have already made dozens of decisions that affect their baby's welfare.

Most parents start out with virtually no preparation save their own experience of being parented. Many hold a new baby for the first time when their own is placed in their arms. The commonest cry heard in the first few weeks after the birth is, 'Why didn't somebody tell me it would be like this?'. It's not only after the birth that parents realize that they need information and skills. Research confirms that expectant parents are interested in preparing for the practical and emotional challenges that a new baby will bring (O'Meara, 1993; Nolan, 1999; Singh and Newburn, 2000).

Starting with yourself

Do you believe that expectant parents are interested in discussing life after birth? On what do you base your beliefs? If you already lead classes, what percentage of the time do you devote to life after birth? What have you heard new parents say they wish they had been better prepared for? What topics and issues do you think about life after birth should be addressed in the antenatal class? At our workshops we regularly ask health professionals what they think should be covered. Common responses include:

feeding, bathing and changing the baby
what to buy for the baby
feelings and emotions
changing relationships
sex and contraception
lochia/after pains
getting enough sleep
accepting offers of help
getting out and about
postnatal exercises
baby checks and immunization
coping with a crying baby
going back to work
baby safety and cot death prevention
what newborn babies need
what type of nappies to use
the blues, postnatal depression
making time for each other
perineal pain
cord care
setting realistic priorities
managing conflicting advice
changing family relationships
postnatal checks
enjoying your baby
where the baby sleeps
affordable childcare
where and when to get help and support

What do you/would you include? If you have limited time, which topics do you think are essential?

As well as deciding what to include, you need to examine your beliefs and attitudes to each topic. For example, how do you feel about women who decide not to breastfeed or who continue to smoke? Do you think that dummies are good or bad? How do you feel about disposable versus reusable nappies? Where should the baby sleep? Do you focus on the mother's needs, or do you discuss the partner's needs as well? How do you react when fathers ask how soon they can have sex after the birth? Is it possible and desirable to get the baby into a routine as soon as possible? How do you react to parents who refuse immunization?

Establishing relevance

When parents first come to class, they are very naturally preoccupied with the prospect of labour and may not appear to be looking further ahead. The key to enabling parents to focus on parenting is to deal with their priorities first. Once you have tackled labour to their satisfaction, they will be more able to consider what comes next. This does not mean leaving all mention of parenthood until later classes; you can prepare the ground by briefly mentioning the baby or some aspect of parenthood in every class.

Practical approaches

There is at least as much that you can say about life after birth as there is about pregnancy and labour, so you may have to be selective. However, you can cover a wide variety of issues in a relatively short space of time by:

- using the approaches to giving information described in Chapter 6
- mentioning babies and parenting in every class
- allocating part of the course to life after birth
- using a variety of active learning techniques.

Mentioning babies and parenting in every class

There are a whole variety of ways in which you can offer parents brief but frequent reminders about babies and parenting. By doing this from the very first class you convey the message that the course is not just about labour and birth and that it is important to think further ahead. Some examples are described below.

Include the baby's experience

Try bringing the baby's point of view into every topic and issue you cover. In this way you remind parents that their baby is affected by everything that happens. What might contractions be like for the baby? What might it be like for the baby to be born? What sort of welcome would help the baby adjust to the bright, noisy, cold world? What are the effects of various procedures on the baby? What is it like for the baby to be monitored? What are the effects on the baby of opiates? An epidural? Entonox?

Think about the messages you send when you talk about babies. No babies are 'it', so use 'he' or 'she' when talking about them, alternating the sex frequently. Handle the doll often, with respect, and as gently as you would a real baby (see Chapter 8).

Draw analogies between current experiences and parenthood

The unpredictable and inevitable nature of labour is like the erratic and continuous needs of a new baby. The disturbed sleep of late pregnancy mirrors broken nights after the birth. The tiredness of early and late pregnancy is like the exhaustion of early parenting. Babies literally come between a couple who want to hug in pregnancy, and are just as intrusive once born. The way nauseated women eat in early pregnancy is similar to the way new babies breastfeed – little and often.

Link skills for labour to parenting skills

The skills you teach for pregnancy and birth can be useful once the baby is born. For example, 'a relaxed parent is more likely to be able to soothe a fretful baby'; 'babies like to be stroked and massaged, and tired parents might enjoy it too!'

Encourage parents to notice their baby's behaviour

Each baby has his or her own patterns of activity and rest. Some are prone to hiccoughs. Some seem to quieten when the father puts his hand on the mother's tummy. A few object when a woman sits for too long. Many become active when the mother relaxes, or startle at loud noises. Start a class with a round asking, 'How has your baby been this week?', or 'Does your baby seem to have any likes or dislikes?'.

Allocating time for life after birth

There is no way that class leaders can equip people for parenthood. Parenthood is a process of evolution. The needs of a newborn baby are different from those of a toddler, a 5-year-old makes different demands from a 10-year-old, and the parents of teenagers may need a whole new set of skills and strategies. However, effective leaders can help parents to make the transition to parenthood by offering a balance of information, practical skills, strategies, and time for reflection. As well as deciding on the information you want to cover, you could consider the following.

Exploring expectations

During pregnancy, expectant parents move from being a child of their parents to being the parent of their child. For better or worse, their expectations and assumptions about parenthood are rooted in their own experience of being parented. Childhood experiences may have been positive or negative, or more usually a combination of the two. When a couple become parents, there are two sets of attitudes and assumptions.

Some may be similar but others may conflict (Daws, 1997). Most couples will benefit from talking and listening to each other so that they can learn about each other's views, feelings and ideas about parenting. They can find out about their partner's expectations and think about how they will share practical chores and baby care as well as finding time for each other.

You can help people to explore and share their ideas and expectations by setting up small groups. You could ask them to discuss what will be good and what will be hard about being a parent, or offer them situation cards (see Chapter 9). The main thing is to get people talking and thinking, and in the process you can offer the relevant information and suggest coping strategies.

Balancing the joys and the challenges

Discussions about parenthood tend to be polarized – parents are either presented with idealized images of relaxed parents holding a beautiful, contented baby, or they are bombarded with dire warnings about how chaotic life will be. You can balance these extremes by giving realistic information coupled with skills and strategies to manage the difficulties, and also by discussing the pleasures – the sense of pride and achievement that parents can feel, the indescribable feel and smell of a newborn baby nestling in one's arms, the joy of the first smile, the satisfaction of watching the baby grow.

Including what babies can do

A great deal is known about what unborn babies can do. From early in the pregnancy, babies can suck, swallow, yawn and show preferences for certain tastes. They can hear, and perceive light. They respond to the mother's activities and moods, and show preferences for different types of music (Chamberlain, 1987, pp. 34, 52; Klaus and Klaus, 1998, p. 3). In other words, unborn babies are alert and aware individuals. (Chapter 11 suggests a way of combining this sort of information with relaxation.)

Babies are born with all senses working. Their facial expressions can convey feelings ranging from pleasure to rage. Contrary to popular belief, babies smile very early – sometimes at birth, if the experience has been gentle (Chamberlain, 1987, p. 54). After some time resting quietly on the mother's chest, a baby is capable of moving towards and finding the mother's nipple unaided. Within hours of birth, babies show a preference for their own mother's odour (Klaus and Klaus, 1998, pp. 10–18).

Immediately after a straightforward birth during which the mother has received little or no medication, newborn babies are often alert and calm for a considerable period of time. They are often extremely interested in the world about them, showing a preference for people rather than other objects. They also respond to human voices, especially those that they have heard before birth. Above all, they are fascinated by faces and will look at them intently. A series of photographs called *Ethan's First Half Hour* (The Children's Project, 2001), taken from a video of a newborn baby's first interactions with his parents, demonstrate quite clearly that not only is the baby fascinated by his parents' faces, but also within the first half hour of his life he can interact. The father holds the baby about 9 inches or 23 centimetres from his face. Then he sticks out his tongue while the baby watches intently, and after a few seconds the baby sticks his tongue out too (Murray and Andrews, 2000; The Children's Project, 2001).

Armed with this sort of information and visual evidence, and given time, peace and quiet after the birth, parents can begin to learn how to communicate with their son or daughter. If they hold the baby about 23 centimetres from their face, support his or her head and pay gentle and sensitive attention, they will probably be rewarded by discovering that their baby is highly responsive and fascinated by them.

Including how babies communicate

Babies are different; some are more relaxed and cuddly than others, some cry more. Some are outgoing, others are easily over-stimulated and need more peace and tranquillity. Even very young babies are extremely expressive. They convey their needs and moods not only by crying but also through their level of eye contact, their facial expressions and body movements. Parents who learn to notice subtle changes in their baby's moods can recognize early signs of distress and prevent it escalating. They can also develop ways of minimizing or avoiding situations that upset their baby (see Murray and Andrews, 2000, for practical approaches).

Teaching practical skills

Many parents want to know how to bath, feed and change their baby. Telling parents that they will be shown these skills when the time comes may satisfy some, but leaves others feeling let down and unprepared. Early discharge from hospital may also leave little time for teaching these skills, and as a result parents may go home feeling ill-equipped and anxious. It may also difficult to include partners after the birth, and they should ideally be taught alongside their partners (see Chapter 13).

If you decide not teach practical skills, you need to explain why and to be confident that parents *will* be shown what to do at another time. If you decide to include these skills in your classes, you need to decide the best way of covering them. This is not always straightforward.

The role of the demonstration baby bath has been questioned. McLoughlin (1996) suggests that watching an expert bath a baby in unfamiliar surroundings and with equipment that may not be available at home may be intimidating rather than empowering. It is quicker and possibly more useful to use a doll to show parents how to wrap and hold a baby in order to wash his face and head, and then how to hold a baby safely while bathing him and lifting him in and out of the water. Then pass the dolls and towels around so that each person can practise (see Figures 15.1 and 15.2).

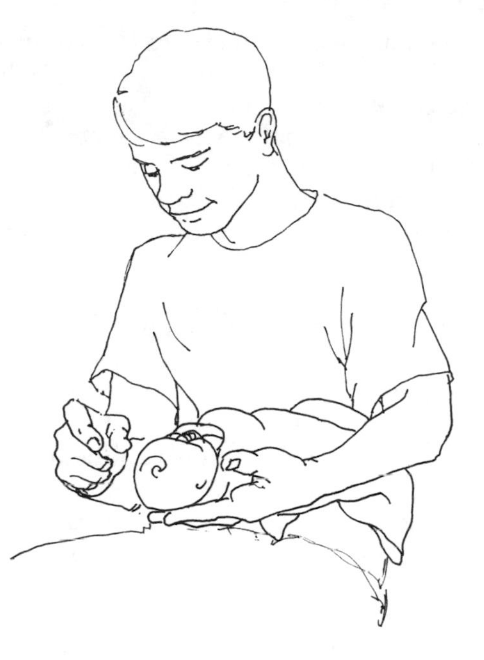

Figure 15.1

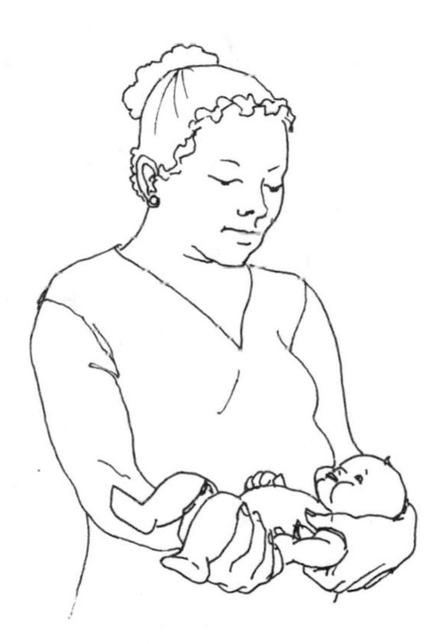

Figure 15.2

Parents need clear, factual and balanced information on the pros and cons of breast- and bottle-feeding and, depending on the choices they make, they also need to know how to position a baby at the breast or how sterilize bottles and make up feeds. However, the UK Baby Friendly Initiative (UNICEF, 2001) states that instructions on how to make up feeds are best given on an individual basis, and that demonstrations in front of a group are unlikely to equip people to make up feeds properly. Contrary to popular belief, the Initiative does not preclude giving factual information about bottle-feeding in a class, so if your unit has achieved Baby Friendly status, the only thing you cannot do is a demonstration of how to make up bottle feeds. It is important to tell parents who decide to bottle-feed that they will be shown how to sterilize and make up feeds individually, and to do everything you can to ensure that this actually happens.

Bringing in a mother, father and new baby

This works best if the baby is under six weeks old, as expectant parents are less likely to identify with an older baby. You will need to take care when choosing whom to ask, as the total focus of the class will be on the parents and, of course, on the baby. The ideal candidates are neither long-winded nor dogmatic. Who will you invite? Someone who had an easy birth, or someone who did not? A mother who is breastfeeding and happy to do so in front of the group, or one who prefers privacy for feeds or is bottle-feeding? A couple, or a mother by herself? It is always wise to see the parents with their baby first to ensure that they are reasonably relaxed and confident. Many years ago one of us had the unfortunate experience of inviting a couple back to an antenatal class during which the father repeatedly demonstrated the strength of his newborn daughter's grasp reflex by suspending her from his thumbs in mid-air!

You will also need to decide how to structure the session. You can run it as an informal discussion, or guide the conversation by asking the parents questions that will encourage them to talk about certain issues. If you choose the latter, include questions that invite the visiting parents to talk about feelings, reactions and coping strategies as well as factual events. If you invite a couple to a couples' class, what role will the partner play? Will you ask both parents to speak to the whole group? Or will you spend some of the time in single sex groups so that the men talk more freely with the new father? (see Chapter 13).

Using active learning techniques

Chapter 9 describes several active learning techniques that are extremely useful for raising issues about life after birth without lecturing. These include *The 24-hour clock, Buttons, Lucky dip, Situation cards* and *Trigger pictures*.

Relating what you teach to the reality of people's lives

All expectant parents need to think about life after birth, but any discussion of parenting needs to be rooted in the realities of people's lives. Social, economic and cultural factors influence people's choices, and what they can and cannot do. The needs and concerns of parents living in poverty or in unsuitable housing are likely to be different from those of parents who are financially secure. The role of the extended family and decision-making about childcare may differ in different cultural and religious groups. Parents with children by previous relationships may be managing more complex lives and relationships. Parents with a disability may need extra help and resources. Try to put yourself in the shoes of the people in your classes, and adapt what you say about life after birth and what you do to include everyone.

Key points

- Research demonstrates that expectant parents are keen to learn about life after birth.
- Parents are more able to focus on life after birth once their needs in relation to labour and birth have been met.
- There is as much to say about life after birth as there is about labour and birth.
- You can cover a large amount of material by:
  - using the approaches to giving information outlined in Chapter 9
  - mentioning babies and parenting in every class
  - using a variety of active learning techniques.
- It is important to talk about both joys and challenges, and to offer coping strategies.
- Raising awareness about what babies can do helps parents begin to relate to and communicate with their babies before and at the birth.

References

Chamberlain, D. (1987). The cognitive newborn. A scientific update. *British Journal of Psychotherapy*, **4**(1), 30–71.

Daws, D. (1997). Family foundations. *New Generation, The Journal of the NCT*, September.

Klaus, M. H. and Klaus P. H. (1980). *Your Amazing Newborn*. Perseus Books.

McLoughlin, A. (1996). Trial by water. *British Journal of Midwifery*, **4**(4), 204–8.

Murray, L. and Andrews, L. (2000). *The Social Baby, Understanding Babies' Communication from Birth*. The Children's Project, CP Publishing (see useful addresses).

Nolan, M. (1999). Antenatal education – where next? *Journal of Advanced Nursing*, **2**(11), 534–8.

O'Meara, C. (1993). An evaluation of consumer perspectives of childbirth and parenting education. *Midwifery*, **9**(4), 210–19.

Singh, D. and Newburn, M. (2000). *Becoming a Father: Men's Access to Information and Support about Pregnancy, Birth and Life with a New Baby*. The National Childbirth Trust.

The Children's Project (2001). *Ethan's First Half Hour* – a series of 10 A4 photographs. The Children's Project.

UNICEF (2001). *Implementing the Baby Friendly Best Practice Standards*. UK Baby Friendly Initiative.

Chapter 16

Planning a course

This chapter discusses issues to consider when planning a course. It describes a way of developing and monitoring your course plan that combines the principles and approaches outlined in previous chapters.

Why plan a course?

Some class leaders plan their courses down to the last detail, leaving little room for manoeuvre. Others argue that if parents are going to be asked what they want, a course plan is unnecessary. We have found the middle way to be the most effective. Parents do not always know what they are going to find useful, so a combination of your agenda and theirs is most likely to meet their needs. Having a plan can also increase your confidence, and helps you to offer a balanced and varied course.

Creating an effective course plan is a bit like planning a journey. Few people set off without working out a route and having some idea of how long the journey is likely to take. However, a pragmatic traveller will also know that, even on the most familiar journey, there may be delays and diversions to negotiate. The same flexibility is needed when planning a course. You need to know what you want to cover, and how and in what order you will tackle each topic. You also need to be willing to follow diversions and respond flexibly to the needs of each group.

Course content

Traditionally, class leaders have either been left to devise their own course content or expected to deliver a predetermined programme. Both have disadvantages. Prescriptive programmes assume that 'one size fits all', and leave class leaders little room to respond flexibly to a group's needs. Sometimes leaders find themselves under pressure to deliver a vast amount in a very limited time. However, when course planning is left entirely to each individual there may be wide variations in style, content and approach, which can result in parents in the same locality having very different experiences. Ideally, class leaders in the same area should plan a core curriculum together. This ensures that all classes will offer the same basic content, but leaves individual leaders the freedom to respond flexibly to the needs of each group.

A shared philosophy

Before you work on content, it is useful to establish a shared philosophy. This helps everyone to define an appropriate style, and to approach course planning from a similar standpoint. We believe that a philosophy for antenatal classes should be founded on the key principles of adult education and of informed choice (see Chapters 2 and 3). Once devised, it should be reviewed regularly and referred to whenever changes to class structure or content are proposed. It could also be given to all new members of staff, whether they lead classes or not, as part of their induction programme.

Defining aims and objectives

Shared aims and objectives also help with the planning. However, it is important to define your aims and objectives with care. They should be consistent with your philosophy and the principles of adult education. They should also reflect what parents are likely to want, and not just the culture and aspirations of class leaders and the organization (see Chapter 2).

Who is the course for?

We suggest that you start by clarifying who your course is for. Is it for:

- women only? If so, are there sessions for fathers? How many? Will you include a fathers-only class? Will you hold a reunion?
- for women and their partners? Are labour supporters invited? Or the mother's mother?
- first-time mothers, with second-timers free to come along if they wish?
- just for primips?
- just for multips?
- for teenagers?
- for women in the last third of their pregnancy, or can they start at any time they wish? Or is there an early pregnancy class for women who are less than 16 weeks pregnant?

What type of course?

You also need to decide whether you are planning for an open or a closed group.

An open group accepts anyone at any class, which means that the group becomes a new entity at every session. In a course of rolling classes you cover a different theme each week, and an open invitation system allows people to join at any point, leaving when their baby arrives or when they feel they have had enough. This offers parents maximum flexibility and encourages those who might otherwise be daunted by classes to have a go. However, it also means that parents are less able to make meaningful contact with others in the group. They may encounter topics in illogical sequences, and are less likely to get all the information and the skills they might need.

The leader, too, has a harder task. You can only run effective, enjoyable open invitation sessions if you are flexible enough to work with any number of people at the drop of a hat, and skilful enough to turn strangers into participants within minutes. It can be done, but it is not easy.

A closed group, on the other hand, offers a complete package. Parents join at the first class, and there is a logical flow of topics over several weeks (pregnancy and the onset of labour in the first week, labour over the next few sessions, then the early days of parenthood). Closed groups offer people an opportunity to get to know each other gradually and to feel safe enough to address more sensitive issues. They can work at their own pace, and you can adapt the course to meet their particular needs. On the negative side, a closed group will only suit those who are able and willing to commit themselves and can plan ahead to fit a course of classes into their lives.

New people can join a closed group successfully at the second meeting if the class knows in advance that another member is expected. After the second week it becomes more difficult, since the group has begun to establish its own unique identity. Some people may drop out after a few sessions because they decide that the course is not for them, or unexpected obstetric events may intervene. Despite these changes, the group usually remains fairly constant because even those not actually present continue to be regarded as members of the group.

Many health professionals feel that closed groups limit attendance and are incompatible with their objective of offering a service to all. Others run closed groups because they feel that offering a quality service (i.e. one that stands the best chance of being effective) is the best way to use precious time and energy. They argue that it makes no sense to judge effectiveness just by totting up the numbers of people who pass through, if nothing significant happens to them along the way.

Still other health professionals take the middle ground. They offer a package of classes that make up a course. They accept everyone who comes and try to give each person an experience that brings them back for more, so that in time the group becomes relatively stable. You will have to work out what would work best for the parents in your area.

Course structure

You also need to decide whether you are designing a set programme or a more flexible course.

A fixed programme consists of a series of classes, each dealing with a separate and predetermined aspect of parent education. For example, one class might be a labour talk, and there may be a relaxation class or classes, a class on pain relief, another on intervention, one on infant feeding, and another on life after birth. This format has advantages for the organization in that parents can slot into another session if they miss one, and it is easier for several leaders to lead different parts of the course. It can also suit parents who might not come to a whole course, but would attend one or two sessions on topics that interest them. However, it also has disadvantages. Parents who choose only one or two sessions may miss out on information and skills that they could have found useful, and they will also miss out on the social side of classes. It is very difficult for the leader or leaders to respond to the immediate needs of the group, and a whole class on the same topic can be rather intense or, in the case of intervention, depressing and off-putting.

A flexible programme combines topics, issues and skills in a much more fluid way. Leaders still plan what they intend to do, but can respond flexibly to the needs of the group and deal with their priorities as they emerge. Physical skills and topics such as intervention and preparation for parenthood can be woven in and linked to each other throughout the course. Time can be used more flexibly, and the leader can ensure that there is a balance of information, physical skills, activities and discussion in each class. Parents can participate in setting the agenda and will want to keep coming, especially if the first class is stimulating and fun. The disadvantage of a flexible programme is that some parents are not able to commit themselves to attending a whole course of classes. In addition, it is harder to find an alternative class for parents who have missed a session, since no two classes are ever likely to cover exactly the same amount of material. Despite these drawbacks, this is the approach we favour.

Class size

Although the basic content of your course will be the same whatever the class size, the numbers attending can influence the type of activities you plan. In addition, the size of your classes will certainly affect timing. The larger the class, the longer it takes to move people around, to help them get to know each other, and to do things like name rounds. We have found that we can only work effectively with a maximum of 24 people.

Time

The length of each class and the number of classes in the course will influence what you can include. This may sound obvious, but we have met many health professionals who have very limited class time and feel they have failed when they cannot cover everything. If you have limited time you will either have to be selective and prioritize, or negotiate to extend the length of classes and/or the number of classes in your course. One way of doing this is to use the course planning exercise below. Using the cards as your focus can help you to remain objective and practical. Lay out your course as it exists now. This will help you to see what is and is not possible in the time you have. You can then show colleagues and managers the plan you have laid out, and demonstrate the limits of what can be covered. If staff shortages make it impossible to extend class time or course length, at least you could agree on what must be covered and what could be left out.

A method of course planning

This method of course planning has been tried and tested by health professionals throughout the UK. It enables leaders to:

- identify essential topics
- plan a logical flow of material and activities
- ensure that there are frequent changes of pace throughout each class
- check that what they plan is likely to fit into the time available
- plan jointly with colleagues
- demonstrate what can be included in the time available and what will have to be cut if, for example, the course is shortened.

If you want to design a course, or review what you already do, you could try this approach on your own. If you and other class leaders want to agree the basic content of classes in your locality, you could plan together. Planning together helps you and your colleagues gain greater mutual understanding and respect. If you share the course with other leaders, you definitely need to plan together even if you are never with the class at the same time (see Chapter 18). Either way you will need several hours of uninterrupted time, ideally on several different occasions. Breaks of hours or even days allow time for reflection, and reduce the chance of your feeling overwhelmed or frustrated by the task. You will, however, need a place where you can be sure that the plan you have started to lay out will not be disturbed by anyone – including the cat!

If you plan in a group you will need to listen to each other with respect, especially when your views differ, and be willing to negotiate. Most people find it helpful to focus on the planning cards (see below) rather than on each other. If anyone gets bogged down in their own professional or personal viewpoint, keep asking, 'What would appeal to parents? What would be the best way of meeting their needs?'.

Begin by asking:

- what do parents need to know to cope with the rest of pregnancy, during labour and in the early weeks of parenthood?
- what do parents need to learn to do with their bodies that would help them during pregnancy and labour, and with the demands of caring for a new baby?
- what hopes and fears, beliefs and ideas would parents benefit from exploring?

Your answers will produce three lists, the first of *information* you could include, the second of *physical skills*, and the third of *attitudes and feelings* – the three components of a balanced course.

Here are the lists that we use to help health professionals plan their course. They include many topics that are traditionally covered in antenatal classes. They will not necessarily include all the topics you think are important, and we are certainly not suggesting that every topic below should or could be included. The list is there to help you to devise your own and to prioritize. In the information section we have broken down large topics such as labour into the different phases and stages in order to be realistic about timing. In the physical skills section we have included a range of ways to teach relaxation to ensure variety. In the attitudes and feelings section we have used open questions, which are likely to generate discussion and reflection.

Information:

Explaining antenatal notes

Role of the midwife and the health visitor

Foetal development

Toxaemia

Maternity benefits

Diet in pregnancy

Dental care in pregnancy

Hormone changes in pregnancy

'Minor' disorders in pregnancy

Overview of the stages of labour

How labour starts

What is a contraction?

Early first stage

Late first stage

Change from first to second stage

Early second stage

Late second stage

Birth of your baby

The third stage

Pain relief – self help

Entonox
Pethidine
Induction and acceleration
Caesarean birth
Episiotomy and suturing
Stillbirth
Preparing for a home birth
Who's who in hospital
The neonatal unit
Sex in pregnancy
Vitamin K
Epidural
TENS
Monitoring
Ventouse and/or forceps
Pethidine
How breastfeeding works
What to take to hospital
Hospital policies and routines
The blues/postnatal depression
Sex after birth and contraception

Physical skills:

Easing backache, pelvic rocking
Pelvic floor exercises
Breathing awareness and relaxation
Visualization with relaxation
Relaxation for living
Positions for first stage
Late first stage positions and breathing
Positions for second stage
Breathing for birth and crowning
Positioning a breastfed baby
Postnatal exercises
Posture and lifting in pregnancy
Recognizing tension versus relaxation
Standing relaxation
Touch relaxation and massage
Relaxation with a painful stimulus
First stage relaxation and breathing
Easing backache in labour
Second stage breathing and pushing
Coping after a Caesarean
Comforting a crying baby
Baby massage

Attitudes and feelings:

Introductions and agenda setting
What will be hard about being a parent?
What do you dislike about pregnancy?
What makes a good parent?
How do you feel about going into labour?
What worries you about labour?
Who do you want with you during labour?
How do you feel about intervention in labour?
What will be good about being a parent?
What do you enjoy about pregnancy?
How has pregnancy changed relationships?
What sort of parents might the baby want?
When will you phone the midwife?
What are your choices for labour?
What pain have you had, and what helped?
Which positions do you find comfortable?

How will you welcome your baby at birth?
What if the baby is not all right?
How do you feel about breastfeeding?
How do you feel about asking for what you want?
What might it be like seeing her in labour?
What help could you give during labour?
How do you feel about leaving work?
How do you feel about taking your baby home?
Where will the baby sleep?
How will this baby fit into the family
What will it be like being 'just a mum'?
What did you feel prepared/unprepared for?
What if things don't go as you hope?
How do you feel about being in hospital?
How do you feel about bottle-feeding?
How do you feel about managing pain?
Will you be there all the time?
How will it feel leaving her in hospital?
How do you feel about going back to work?
How soon would you like to go home?
How could you organize life after birth?
How will you make time for each other?
How could you manage a toddler and baby?
How did your labour go?

Next, you will need sheets of card or paper in three different colours. Cut the sheets into rectangles about the size of a credit card and write each topic or activity on a separate card, using different colours for each group. For example, you could write all the information topics on blue cards, the physical skills on red, and the activities that involve discussion and reflection on green cards.

You will also need cards in a fourth colour on which to indicate the type and number of each class. You could have separate cards for some or all of the following: an early pregnancy class; class one, class two, class three and so on; a couples' course; a women-only course; a fathers' evening (or two); a fathers-only evening; a tour of the maternity unit; and a postnatal reunion. You could also include an infant resuscitation session. Or you could have one card for an all-day class – a labour day.

Now you are ready to start laying out the cards to create your own unique course plan. You need to be methodical, otherwise you may feel overwhelmed. As you select your cards, remember that, on average, *each one will take 10 minutes of class time*, and you will also need to leave time for ice-melting, discussion, reflection, and for what parents want.

Start by laying out the number and type of classes you intend to have in your course. Then take the information cards. We suggest that you begin by selecting all the cards that cover labour. If you lay them out in one long line, you will have a clear outline of a typical 'labour talk'. Add up the amount of time that parents would have to listen to this talk, and compare your total with the average human attention span (see Chapter 3). A labour talk may seem a convenient and an efficient way of delivering information, but in educational terms it is unlikely to be very effective. Instead of telling the story of labour in one omnibus edition, you could tell it in instalments over several weeks. Try laying out the labour cards over two, three or even four weeks. This allows you to intersperse information-giving with relevant physical skills. There will also be time for discussion, reflection and activities in each class.

Now consider the rest of your information cards. You probably have far too many to fit into your course. This means that you will have to be ruthless and decide what is essential. You can do this by:

- including only information topics that are relevant to the people you teach. They are not training to be health professionals, but are preparing for the subjective experience of birth and parenthood
- sticking to what you see as their needs, leaving time to address their wants
- deciding if the information is relevant to parents, given the stage they are at. Will they have received it elsewhere, for example, as a routine part of antenatal care? On these grounds you might eliminate fetal development, dental care, diet, and maternity benefits. These are not trivial matters, but, given the limited time available, you need to choose.
- devising other ways of covering the topic (see Chapter 9).

Now you can start interspersing information cards with physical skills cards. Aim for a logical flow by choosing physical skills that will complement and build on what you have talked about. In a two-hour class, we suggest that you aim to include around two to three short physical skills sessions.

Next add the attitudes and feelings cards. Remember to allow time for introductions and agenda setting, as these are the foundation for interactive learning (see Chapter 5). Look for discussion topics and activities that complement the information and physical skills you have already selected.

This can be a long process. You will probably move some cards several times. You may decide you need an extra class. There is likely to be a lot of discussion and negotiation between members of the group to establish the best spot for certain cards.

When you have chosen your cards, check the timing. Each topic will take at least 10 minutes to do well; a few will take longer. So in a one-hour class you can only include four or possibly five topics or activities if you want to leave time for the group to settle, for people to talk, and for the

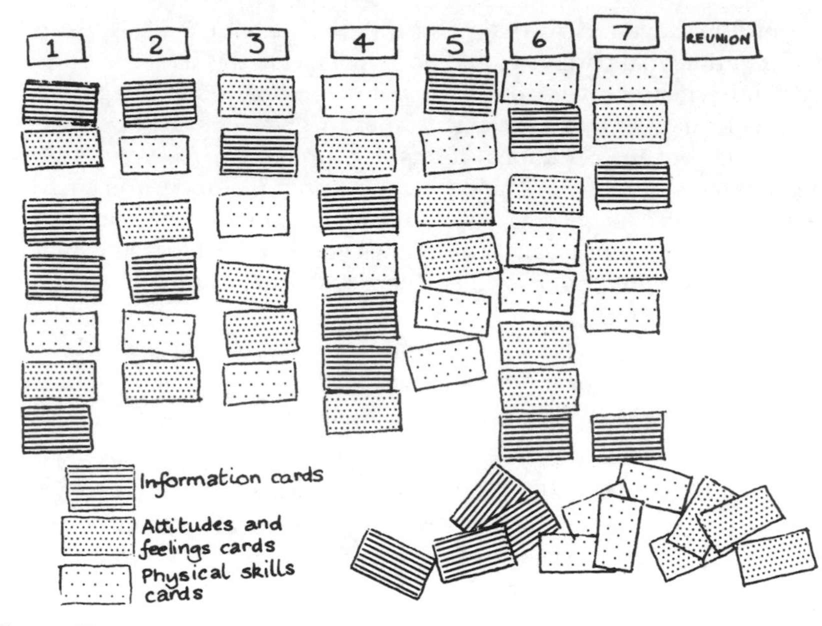

Figure 16.1

unexpected events which always occur. In a two-hour class you might handle around nine cards. The rest must go.

It is often hard to discard topics. You may feel tempted to sneak them back by amalgamating several under one heading (e.g. 'Forceps, monitoring and induction – oh, I'll call that interventions') or by keeping a long list of cards for one class with the idea of spending just a minute or so on each. However, you will serve parents better if you cover a few things well than if you dash through a dozen superficially. Besides, you could never cover everything, even if you had all the time in the world!

Now stand back and look at the colours rather than the words on each card. Is any class top-heavy with one colour? The best sessions offer a mixture of all three activities – information, practising physical skills, and discussing or sharing ideas and feelings. Keep moving the cards until each session contains a balance of all three activities. Finally, look within the session, viewing each column of cards as a chronological record of the class. The best sessions offer the group a new kind of activity every 10 minutes or so. Is this is reflected in colour variation as you move down the line?

Then check that topics are covered in a logical order, and that there is a natural flow of material throughout the course which reflects the way in which parents are likely to encounter the events of pregnancy, labour, birth and parenting.

You now have a grid containing the key topics and activities you want to include in your course, and the order in which you could do them (Figure 16.1). Now you need some practical way of recording your plan.

Table 16.1

COURSE CHECK CARD	LOCATION ______	DATES _____
Ice-melting and agenda setting		
Name round		
Review agenda		
Easing back-ache		
Feelings re going into labour?		
How labour starts		
When will you call the midwife?		

Creating a course check card

Here is a way of recording your plan that also enables you to respond flexibly to individual needs and keep a check on what you have covered with each group you teach.

You need filing cards – A5 size works well. Draw columns leaving small margins between each (Table 16.1). List all the topics and activities in the columns, in the order in which you plan to cover them. You could colour-code them as a reminder to keep changing between information, physical skills, and attitudes and feelings. Leave room on the check card to add the group's wants, and space at the top for the dates and location of the class. If you and your colleagues have agreed a basic course content, you could have standard cards printed.

You need one course check card for each group you teach. At the end of the first class, add any issues that the group wants to cover. After each class, tick off the topics you have covered. We suggest that you keep the card in the room where the class is taught; this means that colleagues who share your class (or who have to take over at short notice) can see what you have planned, what the group wants, and what has been covered. At the end of their class they can tick off the topics they have dealt with, so that on your return you know what remains to be tackled.

Making your own notes

As well as devising a course plan you may want to be able to refer to your own more detailed notes. It can be helpful to have brief reminders for

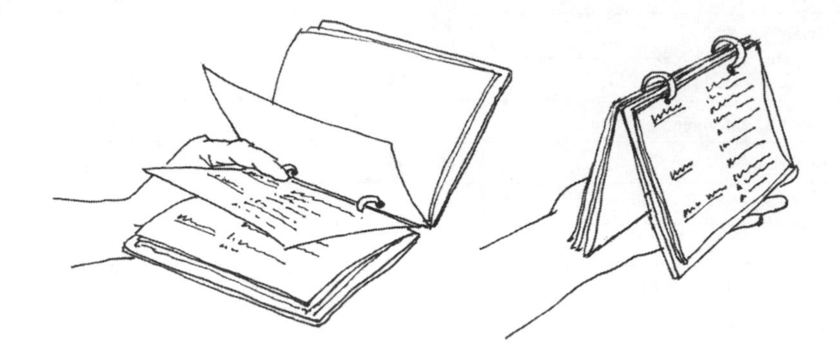

Figure 16.2

activities, the three points you want to make about each topic, and notes on the different types of physical skills you plan to include. Having notes to refer to can be especially helpful if you are new to leading classes, and if you run a flexible programme and want to be able respond to whatever parents bring up.

Working from sheaves of paper can be a bit unmanageable and may not inspire confidence, and a more manageable method is to write brief notes on A5 cards. These can be kept together by punching holes along the top edge and using split rings to bind them together. These look a little like large key rings, but they have a catch and a hinge so that you can open them, thread them through the stack of punched cards and then close them securely. Split rings are available in at least two sizes from most good stationers (Figure 16.2).

If you have read straight through this chapter and feel that it all sounds much too complicated, try it out. You will find that it allows you to convert a swirling mass of ideas and a blank sheet of paper into a coherent course plan.

Key points

- Effective course planning helps to ensure that classes are varied and that essential topics are covered.
- A shared philosophy helps staff in the same locality to plan together.
- Before starting to plan, it is important to define who the classes are for, whether the classes will be open or closed, and whether the design will be fixed or flexible.
- A method of course planning is described in this chapter.
- A course plan should be used flexibly so that parents' needs are accommodated as they arise.
- A course check card helps class leaders to keep track of what has been covered during the course, especially when different classes are led by different leaders.

Chapter 17

Meeting different needs

Expectant parents represent a cross-section of the population. This chapter looks at ways of responding to possible variations in need, and discusses how to reach people who do not come to classes.

Expectant parents have a great deal in common, but for a variety of reasons some have additional needs. For example, they may already have children; they may be expecting twins or more; they may be unsupported, have a female partner, be very young, or belong to a conservative cultural or religious group.

You can either encourage everyone to come to existing classes, work one-to-one, or run separate sessions for specific groups. Running standard classes and inviting everyone regardless of need may be the only option if numbers are low or resources are limited. However, some people will not come either because they fear that they will not fit in or because they do not think classes will meet their needs. If people with differing needs do come to existing classes, it is important to ensure that their needs are met and that everyone is integrated into the group. If two or more people in the class have similar needs, perhaps, for example, because they are expecting their second or third child, it is almost always helpful to set up small groups so that they can discuss their own particular perspectives while the rest of the group focuses on other things. Alternatively, you could include a single session specially designed for parents who, for example, already have children.

Sometimes there will be enough people – for example, teenagers, people expecting second or subsequent babies, or women of a minority culture or religion – to run classes just for them. You can focus entirely on what they want, and they can share experiences, exchange support and learn from each other.

Starting with yourself

Your own attitudes and assumptions will not only influence the way you relate to people with differing needs but will also affect your ability to model inclusiveness for the rest of the group. Everyone makes assumptions about other people; some are conscious but most are not. Guirdham (1990) uses the analogy of an iceberg, with conscious assumptions being the visible tip, while the unacknowledged majority lie submerged and invisible, ready to cause damage to anyone who bumps into them! Assumptions are an unreliable basis for action, and especially for relating to people, so it is vital to check them out. What do you believe and think about teenagers, parents with a disability, lesbians, or the different religious and cultural groups in your area? On what do you base your beliefs? Are your sources reliable? Is what you have heard likely to apply to everyone in that group regardless of origin, education, social situation and personality?

Being inclusive

Whether you incorporate everyone into mainstream classes, work one-to-one or run special classes for different groups, there are several principles that apply.

- The things expectant and new parents have in common more than balance out their differences.
- The individual is the expert on what she or he needs and wants, so ask. This must be done with respect and tact, and in ways that preserve people's confidentiality. This is especially important for people who experience discrimination, racism or homophobia on a regular basis. It is up to them to decide what they want you and the rest of the group to know.
- Nobody likes to feel marginalized, so model respect, and make sure that everything you say and do includes everyone and avoids singling anyone out.
- Do everything you can to ensure that individuals are treated equitably by other participants. You cannot change other people's beliefs and attitudes, but you can influence behaviour in your group – for example by giving everyone equal time, and setting ground rules and ensuring that they are observed.
- Find out from those who have attended your classes how you could improve what you offer. It might be better to do this on a one-to-one basis.

Parents expecting second and subsequent babies

Parents who already have children are often invited to attend classes run primarily for first-time parents. Their presence can be enriching, adding realism and colour, which first timers often appreciate. Experienced parents can benefit too, especially if they have not attended classes before or if it is some years since they last gave birth. However, there can also be drawbacks. If the primary focus is the needs of first-time parents, it is all too easy to neglect the additional needs of 'multips'. Occasionally an experienced parent uses the class as an opportunity to debrief a traumatic experience. The leader is then faced with the difficult task of offering appropriate support to the person who needs to debrief and at the same time attempting to give the first timers a more balanced view of what is likely to happen to them.

In a course designed specifically for experienced parents you can focus entirely on their needs. Experienced parents usually know what they want from classes. Most need to talk about their last labour(s) before they are ready to focus on the next. Only a lucky few will have done this, leaving the rest full of undigested birth stories just waiting to be told. This 'debriefing' is more effective if it is systematic. If each person is offered the chance to be heard, he or she can begin to make sense of what happened and share feelings and experiences. In a small group (not more than six) you could give each person a predetermined amount of time to speak while the others listen without interrupting. Even five minutes of uninterrupted attention, during which no one advises, judges or sidetracks with their own comments or stories, can be a powerful experience. In a large group, break them into twos or threes (fours if it is a couples' class) and divide the time equally. This encourages the more silent to speak, and ensures that people unused to listening do not have too many stories to take in. You can start them off, keep them focused, and elicit their current needs by asking each person, 'How did your last labour(s) go? What went well? What would you like to be different this time?'.

Now and again you will encounter someone who had a childbearing loss or whose experiences were very traumatic. This will need sensitive handling, and those concerned may need more time or more skill than can be offered in class. You could either offer them individual attention later or refer them for specialized help.

As well as looking backwards, this group will want to plan ahead. Experienced parents often say that the main benefit of going to classes is having time away from their busy lives to acknowledge this baby and this impending birth. They are also likely to want to think about how this baby will fit into the family. Some may be concerned about who will look after the first child so that the father can be with the mother during labour. Above all, many parents are anxious about how they will make space in their lives and their hearts for another child when the first seems so all-absorbing. They may be keen to discuss sibling rivalry, normal reactions to a new baby, juggling the needs of two or more children, and possible ways to ease the transition from only child to big brother or sister.

Parents expecting twins or more

Parents who are expecting more than one baby have a great deal in common with all other parents. However, they nearly always have additional concerns. They may be shocked by the prospect of more than one baby, and worried about the practical and financial implications. They are also likely to find themselves receiving extra attention both from the medical profession and from society as a whole. Some attention is welcome, but it can also be intrusive and unhelpful. The reactions of friends and relatives, especially grandparents, are often polarized. Some greet the news with pure delight, while others give dire warnings about what hard work it will be. It is important to help parents find a balanced view, to help them develop their own coping strategies, and to focus on them as individuals and not just on the fact that they are expecting more than one child.

Parents expecting twins or more are more likely to be anxious about the welfare of their babies and about the birth. Their choices about management are often limited, intervention is highly likely, and they also face an increased risk of premature labour and having a baby in special care. Classes can help them prepare for these possibilities and give them a chance to think about how they will deal with them.

They will certainly want to think ahead about life after birth. They may need time to explore their feelings about the prospect of having more than one baby, as well as thinking about how they will manage to feed and care for two or more, get enough sleep and do the essential household chores. Couples will need to think about how they can co-operate, work as a team, and minimize the extra strain that caring for twins or more can put on their own relationship.

Having contact with people in the same boat is reassuring. If at all possible, arrange for parents expecting more than one baby to meet with each other. Contact with parents who are already have twins or triplets is useful, and can help expectant parents prepare for the realities of life after birth. You could also pass on information about local support networks and clubs for parents of twins, triplets and more babies.

Some parents who are expecting more than one baby may have had fertility treatment. They have already had a long and traumatic journey and have had to cope with alternating despair and hope. Although some expectant parents are euphoric, others are anxious and experience mixed feelings when the realities of pregnancy and parenthood are not quite as they imagined. Parents in this situation may need extra support; however, in the class, it is important to respect people's confidentiality. Although many people are happy for others to know they have had fertility treatment, some see it as a very private and personal matter, and a few fear that they will be stigmatized (Bryan, 2000).

Parents with multiple families

An increasing number of couples have complex families. A survey of 817 expectant and new fathers found that one in ten men had a child or children by a previous partner (Singh and Newburn, 2000). The baby may be her first but his third, or her second and his first. When one partner is experienced and the other is not, they are out of step with each other. The shadow of former relationships may hang over this birth (will she do the same as X? Will I measure up to Y?). In addition, at least one partner and his or her children have experienced loss as a result of separation, divorce or death (Braun, 1998). The issues and the sensitivities of the people involved are complex.

You may know the history of a particular couple. However, it may be treated as secret information, a reflection of how problematic many people find this pattern of parenthood. Some parents might let the group know how this baby fits into their family, but until they do so it is essential to respect their confidentiality. If you don't know, don't make assumptions. Even in a group where everyone looks like the stereotypical family, there may be some people who face these issues. Couples in this situation may need extra encouragement to remember that each birth and each baby is unique. They may also need time to consider the effects of the new baby on existing children who already face the additional complexities of belonging to a multiple family.

Teenagers

Whatever their age, teenagers have all the characteristics of adult learners (see Chapter 3). If they are treated equally and with complete respect, very young women can often benefit and gain confidence from being in an ordinary class. However, many do not come. If this is true in your area, it may make sense to plan a course specifically for them.

Starting with yourself

Start by reviewing your own attitudes and feelings. Are teenage parents irresponsible or stupid? Do they get pregnant in order to be housed? Are they more likely to be promiscuous or to abuse drugs? Are they incapable of being good parents? Are they always unsupported by the baby's father? Should they have terminated the pregnancy? Should they give the baby up for adoption? Have some of them made a conscious decision to have their baby, and might they be as keen as any other parent to give their child the best and most loving care? Some of these comments could be relevant to some teenagers in some circumstances, but will certainly not apply to everyone (Baker, 1999).

In addition to the principles already outlined earlier in this chapter, you may find it helpful to consider the following.

After the birth

What makes good classes for teenagers work – that is, your friendly, informal, supportive approach – also makes them hard to give up unless there are other suitable groups into which a young mother can 'graduate'. Many leaders who run classes for teenagers welcome young parents back into the group after the birth. New mothers gain confidence and self-esteem from sharing their experiences, and expectant parents learn from being with new babies. Also, young mothers remain accessible to receive further help with parenting.

Including grandmothers

Health professionals who work with teenagers and their mothers sometimes say that the very young mother's mother can be as needy as her daughter. If both are welcome the girl may get little space for herself, as her own mother might either speak for them both or use the opportunity to address her own concerns. Yet excluding grandmothers could shut out the only support many young women have. One solution is to run parallel groups, sometimes all meeting together for common issues, and sometimes splitting into generation groups to consider issues and feelings with others 'in the same boat'.

Including young fathers

Whilst many pregnant teenagers are unsupported by the baby's father, there are young men who want to be involved. Young fathers need encouragement as well as opportunities to find out about birth and parenting and to talk about their concerns and feelings. Find out if the father is at all involved, and offer him a specific invitation to the group (Figure 17.1).

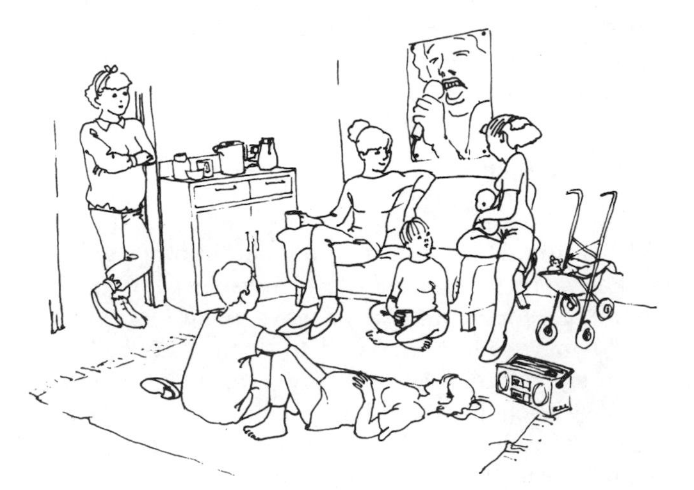

Figure 17.1

Parents of minority cultural and religious groups

Starting with yourself

It is not only minorities who have an ethnicity and a culture – that is, 'ways of doing and viewing things' – we all do. You may be as unaware of the rules, taboos and assumptions of your own culture and ethnic group as you are of the gravity that holds you to your chair. However, you will work better with people who belong to other groups if you are aware of what is considered acceptable and normal in your own culture and in the culture of your workplace.

For example, in the UK it is customary to have regular antenatal checks, to have a baby in hospital and be cared for by strangers, and to be sent home hours or a couple of days after the birth. It is common for fathers to be present at the birth. Going to antenatal classes is accepted practice for many people. Women are expected to be autonomous and independent, and to make their own decisions. However, these 'customs' may be unfamiliar, alien or in some cases unacceptable to people of certain minority cultural and religious groups.

What have you heard about the minority groups in your area? Are the sources reliable? Is what you have heard likely to apply to everyone in that group? If you yourself belong to a minority cultural or religious group, how do you feel about people from your 'group' who do things differently from the way you do them? How do you feel about the other minority groups in your area?

Acknowledging individuality

Within all major religions there are different denominations and differences in belief and practice. A woman who identifies herself as Jewish may be secular – that is, she has Jewish heritage and culture, but is not religious. Alternatively, she may be religious and observe some, many, or all of the Jewish laws. So there is no guarantee that the things you have heard or read about an ethnic or religious group will apply to any particular individual. People outside a culture or religion tend to ask general questions such as, 'What do Sikhs do about birth?'; 'How do Filipinos feel about modesty?'; 'Do Muslim men want to attend the birth?' Tempting though generalizations may be, consider how would you react to the same kind of query about your group. Do health professionals prefer baths or showers? What do mothers in Guildford, Aberdeen or Belfast want for their sons?

People of different cultures who have been brought up and educated in this country straddle two cultures and are likely to be familiar with the British health care system. Those who came to the UK as adults, and especially those who face language barriers, may find the system of health care baffling, confusing and alienating.

Identifying needs

Cultural and religious factors affect a whole variety of issues that are relevant to childbearing and parenting, and the cultural norms of the majority may not apply to people of minority cultures or religions. For example, attitudes to family relationships, gender roles, decision-making and responsibility may be significantly different. Traditions or taboos relating to food, sexual matters, childbearing and baby care may also differ. Rules about washing, modesty, dress codes, hair care, jewellery or religious observance could also be different from those of the majority and from your own (Schott and Henley, 1996).

Formulating the right questions

The key to finding out what people are likely to need is to ask them. However, you need to frame your questions carefully. Broad questions such as 'do you have any cultural or religious needs' are hard to answer, especially for people who do not know what classes involve. Specific questions are more likely to elicit helpful information, especially if you make it clear that you are asking in order to meet their needs. So you could explain how classes are usually organized and then ask, for example, if the dates and times are suitable; if they have any requirements in relation to food and drink; how they feel about birth videos, or about being in a group with men.

Cross-cultural communication is not easy, and there are bound to be misunderstandings from time to time. Most people will be forgiving if you admit to your mistakes or lack of knowledge, especially if they believe that you are genuinely doing your best to meet their needs. Many will be delighted to enlighten you. However, bear in mind that people may not know why they do or do not do certain things, any more than you could give reasons for the way you do things.

The questions you need to ask will be different for different cultural and religious groups. Here are some common themes to consider when planning and designing your classes.

Festivals

Before fixing class dates, find out about the religious and cultural festivals (including the Sabbath) that are observed by people in your locality. For example, for observant Jews the Sabbath runs from sundown on Friday to sundown on Saturday. No work or travel is permitted on the Sabbath, so on Fridays women tend to be very busy with Sabbath preparations, which must all be completed before sundown. Saturday is also the Sabbath for Seventh Day Adventists, while Friday is the Muslim day for prayer. The dates of most religious festivals vary from year to year as, like Easter, many are fixed according to the lunar calendar (SHAP, 2000). It is also useful to know a bit about different festivals. Is a festival happy or sad, a feast or a fast? Is it a time of prayer, for being with family, or for community celebrations? Or do people carry on everyday activities with some adaptations – as, for example, the fast of Ramadan, during which Muslims only eat and drink during the hours of darkness?

Relationships between men and women

In some cultures and religions women do not traditionally mix with men outside their own family, so mixed classes may be inappropriate. Some women may remain completely silent if a man is present. In some conservative cultures and religious groups, women tend to defer to their husbands or to senior family members, at least in public. They may be unused to going out by themselves or to making decisions on their own.

Modesty

In conservative cultures and religious denominations modesty is often an important issue, especially for women. For some this means wearing clothes that are high necked and either cover their arms and legs completely, or cover their arms to below the elbow and their legs to well below the knee. Some women keep their hair covered, especially in public and in the presence of men outside their own family.

Some people consider any mention of intimate body parts immodest, especially in a mixed-sex group. Sometimes finding an appropriate word is a problem. In some Asian languages, for example, there are no socially acceptable words for parts of the body between the waist and the knees. Some people may be offended and distressed by some of the charts, diagrams, videos and posters that are used in hospitals and clinics. Women of many communities have told us of the embarrassment and humiliation they felt watching birth films, especially with other women's husbands present.

Concepts of politeness

Cultural beliefs about appropriate body space, gestures, levels of eye contact and touch vary enormously, and are the hardest to change when adapting to a different culture. For example:

- downcast eyes may be a sign of respect and deference
- pointing the soles of the feet towards another person is very offensive in some cultures
- some people may be offended if you hand them something with your left hand or offer it to them on their left-hand side. This is because in some cultures people reserve their left hand for unclean activities, such as cleaning themselves after using the lavatory, and their right for clean activities such as eating.

Food

People who observe cultural or religious requirements in relation to food may prefer to drink from disposable cups and to be offered biscuits that do not contain any animal fat. Herbal teas may be welcomed by people who avoid stimulants such as tea and coffee.

Finding out

You may now be thinking that you are entering a minefield, and certainly there is a great deal to consider. However, you do not have to know everything, and nor do you have to get everything right. Most people are very forgiving as long as they feel you have their interests at heart. Many are very willing to explain and make suggestions. All you have to do is ask.

A good place to start is with parents who already know and trust you. If there is a sizeable population of a particular group in the neighbourhood, you could approach specialist advice centres, cultural associations or religious groups. The best people to help are those with one foot in each culture – yours and theirs. If you find such a bridge, look after the person well – he or she is your best asset. However, be aware whatever you learn will not apply to everyone from that group or community.

Integrated classes

Having identified the potential issues, it is perfectly possible and indeed enriching for all those involved to have parents from a wide variety of cultural and religious backgrounds in the same class. However, remember that some people may be happy to discuss their differing traditions or rituals while others may not, or may not want to be appear different from others in the class.

If you incorporate people from minority cultures and religions in mainstream classes, you will need to accommodate differing needs with tact and discretion. For example, how would you teach touch relaxation or massage if you had an orthodox Jewish couple in the class? They may not wish to touch each other in public, and the husband may not touch his wife during labour once she has had any vaginal blood loss. The way babies are welcomed at birth varies for different groups. Male circumcision will be an issue for some. How do you feel about it, and would you mention it in your classes?

If you have several people from the same group in your course, it may be helpful to offer them time together whilst the rest of the class focuses on another topic. Alternatively, you might offer them a session on their own to discuss specific issues that are important to them. This has the additional advantage of also offering you a deeper insight into their needs and perspectives.

Separate classes

If parents from minority groups do not come to existing classes, or if there are people who do not speak much English, separate and specifically

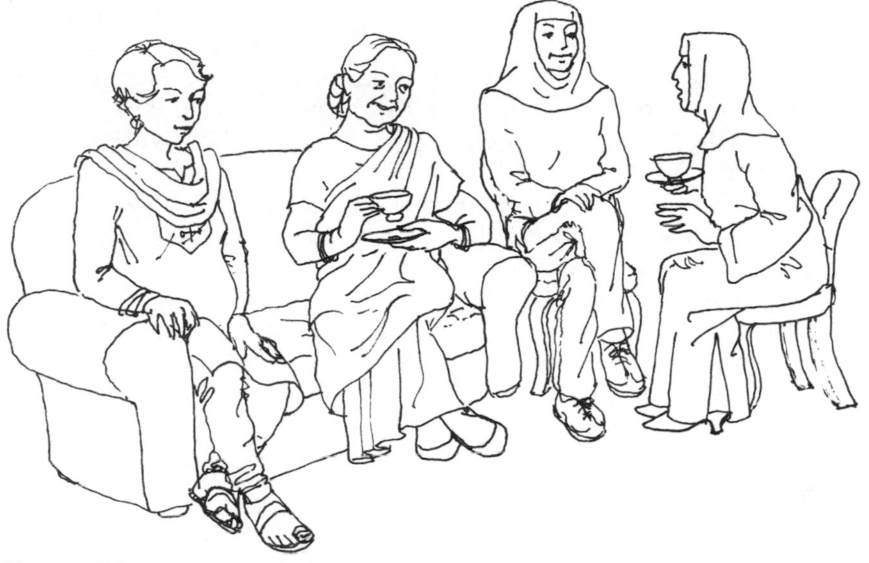

Figure 17.2

designed courses may be the answer. In addition to the principles outlined above, you may find it helpful to consider the following.

Invite the right people to the class. In some conservative cultures, mothers and mothers-in-law are likely to be an important influence on expectant and new mothers. Inviting older women to the class may be a good way of increasing attendance and of informing the people who make the decisions. Women-only sessions are likely to be more acceptable to those who lead largely segregated lives (Figure 17.2).

Working across language barriers

Women who speak a little English

People frequently understand far more than they can say, and the following strategies can maximize your effectiveness.

- Plan what you want to say carefully.
- Choose everyday words, and avoid specialist terms and jargon.
- Listen for the words the parents use (and therefore know) and use them.
- Speak slowly and try not to get louder.
- Take one issue at a time, and present things in a logical order.
- If it is important to check understanding, avoid questions that invite a 'yes' answer. 'Yes' is one of the first words anyone learns in a foreign language, but it does not necessarily signal understanding. 'Yes' can mean: 'Yes I am listening but I am too tired and confused to take in

what you are saying, though I know you mean well,' or, 'Yes I am embarrassed that I don't understand and I don't want to put you and the rest of the class to any more trouble'. Instead, try asking the participants to tell you what they think will happen or what they will do – for example, 'What will you do if your waters break?'; 'When will you bring your baby to the clinic?'.
- Don't be too ambitious. Communicating across a language barrier is tiring and stressful for both sides, but particularly for the person who is trying to understand another language.
- Learn some simple words and phrases in the client's language. One or two words or phrases learned from clients or from a phrase book can help to break down the barriers. It demonstrates empathy, and puts you on a more equal footing.

Working with a professional interpreter

Interpreters for antenatal classes should always be female, since modesty is likely to be an important issue for many of the women who do not speak English, You can work with an interpreter either with you leading the group and the interpreter bridging the cultural and language gap, or as a team, each offering what you do best. In some places the health professional acts more as a consultant, helping the interpreter to gain the knowledge and group skills needed to run the class and then standing by as a resource for technical questions and ongoing support. However you work with your interpreter, doing it well will require skill, patience and a good deal of practice. The key element in an effective working relationship with an interpreter is a clear understanding of what each of you wants from the other and an agreement about aims and objectives.

Interpreting from one language to another is never straightforward. No two languages use exactly the same grammatical structures, or express things in the same way. What seems like the same word rarely means quite the same thing in another language. The more different the roots and structure of two languages – for example, Bengali and English – the more difficult the translator's job. *Her task is to translate meanings rather than words*, and this takes time, skill and concentration. You can help her by:

- making your meaning as clear as possible, using plain language and avoiding jargon
- allowing enough time – one sentence in English may need a much longer explanation in another language, especially if the topic is unfamiliar to the client
- pausing frequently to allow the interpreter to translate – if you say too much at once, something may be forgotten or get left out.

Managing good relationships

Relationships and mutual trust are more complicated but no less important when you are working across a language barrier and with an interpreter. You can promote good three-way relationships by:

- asking the interpreter to introduce herself and explain her role, then introducing yourself to the group through the interpreter
- behaving as normally as you can. Look at the participants when you speak and when the interpreter is speaking, and make it clear through your body language that they, not the interpreter, are the focus of your attention
- recognizing that the interpreter also plays an important role as advocate for the participants
- being aware that the interpreter receives the direct impact of participants' anxieties and fears, and may need your support to deal with these and respond constructively
- taking time with the interpreter beforehand and afterwards, making it clear that you value her skills and experience, and discussing how best to work together.

Working with an untrained interpreter

Some women bring someone with them to interpret. This is never ideal, and if the interpreter is male, which is likely, he may inhibit the other women in the class. You can minimize some of the difficulties if you:

- include the interpreter in your introductions so that everyone present understands his or her role
- listen carefully to their English and, if it is patchy, simplify your language, keep your sentences short and use words that you hear them use
- be patient. It is difficult and distracting to have someone talking to one woman throughout the class, but without the interpreter she would lose out completely.

Communicating across a language barrier is frustrating, but it is worth doing the best you can. It is even more stressful and exhausting for those people on the other side of the barrier, and they have much more to lose than you. (For more information on communicating across language barriers and finding interpreters, see Sanders, 2000.)

Parents with a disability or chronic illness

If you are faced with the prospect of having a person with a physical disability, learning difficulties, or concurrent physical or mental illness in your class, your first thought might be to search the literature or contact relevant organizations. This may well be helpful. However the most expert source of information on their needs is the person themselves. People with a disability or illness have plenty of experience and know what suits them, so ask. This may be hard if you feel that, as the professional, you are expected to have all the answers. However, people would much rather *tell* you what they need and want. This puts them in control, maintains their independence, and respects their knowledge and dignity. It also helps you to avoid mistakes and to be more likely to meet their needs.

Starting with yourself

Keep assessing your own attitudes and prejudices, as these will seep into everything you say and do. Almost without exception, babies born to parents with a disability are both planned and wanted (National Childbirth Trust, 1985). Can you welcome their decision? People with physical disabilities are used to devising ingenious ways of managing the demands of everyday living, and they will do the same in parenthood. Do you believe in their ability to care for their child? Every parent has more abilities than disabilities, and also has a great deal in common with other parents. Although some things will, of necessity, be different, nobody wants to be defined or related to solely on the basis of their disability or illness.

Identifying needs

It may be helpful to meet the person concerned before the classes start so that together you can work out how to meet his or her needs, and find out if the person wants to tell the rest of the group about the disability or illness. You will also need to think about every aspect of your classes from this person's point of view. For example will access to the building, the room and lavatories be easy or difficult for a person with limited mobility? Are the chairs suitable? How will you have to adapt the activities and the physical skills you teach? Parents with a visual impairment are likely to need hands-on alternatives to videos, demonstrations and visual aids, and will need Braille or taped versions of any handouts you use (Mumford and Bhavsar, 1993). Some people with hearing loss lip-read, so you will need to find out what speed to talk at and ensure that they can see your face clearly whenever you are talking. Alternatively, they may want to bring a signer with them (Figure 17.3). How can you simplify information giving, teaching aids, activities and handouts for people with learning difficulties?

Some parents may want to discuss how their disability or medication might affect their pregnancy and labour and, conversely, how pregnancy and birth might affect their condition. For example, some disabilities, illnesses and medication can limit choices about delivery, analgesia and

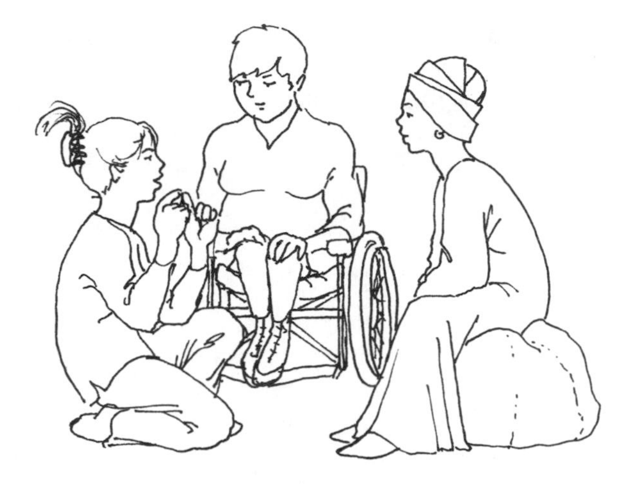

Figure 17.3

infant feeding. Some chronic illnesses are exacerbated by pregnancy, while others tend to go into remission but may flare up again after the birth (Carty, 1995). Without good collaboration between specialists, people with a disability or chronic illness can fall between two stools – their usual doctor may know little about obstetrics, and obstetricians may not know much about the disability or illness.

Parents with learning difficulties may need extra care and reassurance. They are often dependent on others, and may have had poor care in the past or been open to abuse. They may feel especially vulnerable during pregnancy, and may be frightened that they will receive poor, unsupportive care during the birth. This is especially likely if they have not received constructive support and clear, simple information about what will happen and how they might feel (Maternity Alliance, 1999, pp. 16–21). Their needs are more likely to be met in classes specially designed for them, since other parents can have low levels of tolerance to people with learning difficulties (Maternity Alliance, 1999, pp. 7–10).

You do not have to have the answers, but you may be the best person to find sources of information and support. Finding out about local community and voluntary support networks will give you an opportunity to learn more, and will enable you to offer these resources to people who do not already know about them.

Becoming an advocate

Once you have discovered an individual's needs and preferences, you could, with their agreement, act as an advocate, passing on suggestions to clinical care staff. For example, you might let labour ward staff know if a deaf woman uses sign language or lip-reads, and what she needs to be able to communicate effectively; ask postnatal ward staff to organize storage space for a wheelchair or an artificial leg within easy reach of the bed; let them know how a woman who is blind likes to orientate herself and find her way around; and negotiate to allow a women with a chronic illness to maintain or at least share control over her medication. Don't try to anticipate what will be helpful. Keep asking the individuals concerned – they are the real experts.

In class

Continuity, safety and trust are paramount for people who are coping with illness or disability. Constantly having to adjust to different leaders and repeatedly having to explain the same things to each one is stressful, exasperating and exhausting. Having the same person for every session is essential. You need to allow extra time, as some things may take longer than usual. Topics such as disability and screening for abnormality need to be handled with care and sensitivity, as some disabled parents may have more positive attitudes to disability than the other parents in the class (Disability, Pregnancy and Parenthood International, 2001, personal communication).

It may not be easy to balance a disabled person's need to be like everyone (except in the few areas where extra help is obviously needed) with your desire to tailor everything to fit his or her particular situation. Check regularly that you are getting it about right, either as part of a more general feedback session, or in a quiet aside during a coffee break.

Parents who are lesbian

Homophobia and myths about lesbians are deeply rooted in society and in institutions. Lesbians are usually defined solely by their sexuality and portrayed as being unnatural. This affects the way that lesbian women, particularly those who are pregnant, are viewed and treated (Wilton, 1999). It also explains why some women remain invisible, choosing not to go public about their sexual orientation and their relationships.

Starting with yourself

Do you assume that all pregnant women are heterosexual? How do you feel about people in same-sex relationships? When you hear the word lesbian, do you think primarily about sex or about a loving relationship? What do you think about lesbians as parents of boys and of girls? On what do you base your views – verifiable fact, experience, media portrayals or hearsay? If the prospect of having lesbian women in your class makes you uneasy, ask yourself why – what difference does it actually make?

'The lesbian label ... tells you little about the woman who claims it'. It does not tell you the type of sexual activity she engages in. She may or may not have a partner. She may or may not intend to share parenting with her partner. She may or may not maintain contact with the biological father (Saffron, 1999). For many women, being a lesbian is not centred on sex but on a loving relationship with another woman (Kitzinger, 1985). Parents who are lesbian have, by definition, planned the pregnancy and given a great deal of thought to how they will conceive and care for their baby. Partners in a long-term relationship have also had to decide which of the two will bear the child.

In class

The fear of homophobia may prevent women from disclosing their sexual identity and lifestyle. The important thing is to provide a warm, inclusive and respectful environment in which the woman (and her partner) can choose how much they want to disclose to you and the group (Saffron, 1999). If a woman has told you that she is a lesbian you will need to use tact and discretion, especially if she has not told the group. How can you ensure that lesbian parents get the information they need without having to 'come out'?

Although many of their needs are similar to those of the majority, some aspects of parent education classes need adjusting. Think about everything you say and do in your classes. Subtle changes could make all the difference. Talk about partners rather than fathers. Review your teaching aids, posters and leaflets. Do they all imply that a partner is always male? What will partners have in common regardless of gender? What needs and feelings might they share during pregnancy, labour and during the transition to parenthood? What might be different? Think about how you could include the information that lesbian women need without drawing attention to them.

For example, how you will talk about sex? Mentioning the fact that some people believe that sexual intercourse might trigger an overdue labour is not enough. You need to be more specific, and discuss not only the possible effects of semen on the cervix (which is of course only relevant to heterosexuals), but also the possible effects of nipple stimulation and orgasm. Information about sex after birth is important for everyone, but in a few respects the needs of lesbians differ from those of heterosexuals (Wilton, 1996). For example, everyone is likely to want to know when they can have sex after the birth, and they all need to know that many new mothers have a sore perineum and find that sexual desire and vaginal lubrication is reduced for a time. However, the way in which you offer practical tips may imply that you are talking only about penile penetration. You can be more inclusive if, instead of saying 'it is important to choose positions for sexual intercourse that keep pressure off the woman's perineum', you say 'many new mothers find any pressure on the perineum uncomfortable in the first few weeks'. Contraception is important for heterosexuals but not for lesbians, so how will you introduce the topic?

As always, the best sources of information and insights are the people concerned. If you develop a good relationship with lesbian parents, ask them what you could do to make your classes more inclusive and relevant. However, intimate questions about lifestyle, sexual identity or sexual practices are inappropriate and intrusive (Saffron, 1999). They are also discriminatory, since it is highly unlikely that heterosexuals would be asked such questions in relation to parent education.

Local gay and lesbian health and community networks and organizations such as Pink Parents (see useful addresses) may be good sources of information for you and for the lesbian women you teach.

Parents who do not come to classes

Women whose needs are least likely to be met by standard antenatal classes are young, single, working-class women, women who are homeless, those who have a physical disability or a mental health problem, drug users, those who speak little or no English, women of minority cultural and religious groups, and asylum seekers. These are also the women who are likely to have fewer resources, greater need for support and poorer outcomes, and who are less able to access information and manage the health care system (Schott and Henley, 1991; Cliff and Deery, 1997). Since standard provision does not meet everyone's needs, a more flexible and responsive approach is needed.

Starting with yourself

People who are reluctant to attend classes often have plenty of experience of prejudice, stereotyping, judgmental attitudes and pressure to change. Not surprisingly, they tend to avoid situations where they might receive more of the same. Even the most well-meaning class leaders can unintentionally convey attitudes that are off-putting, alienating, and form an invisible but powerful barrier. When we ask class leaders 'Why do you want them to come?', the responses are often very revealing and sometimes disarmingly frank. Some are tongue-in-cheek, but are no less telling for that. Here are some samples drawn from two groups of 24 class leaders in 1999:

We feel they should

To reduce their stress

To increase their self-esteem

To reduce fear

It makes our job easier

They need to be taught about labour and parenting

To increase their social skills

To learn about the culture of the NHS

To help make them better parents

They need help

To keep us in a job
So they don't feel alone
So that they can get to know us
To enable informed choice
To prevent postnatal depression
To help them to have a broader view

To dispel myths about us, pregnancy and parenting
To get support and to network
So that we can get to know them and their partners
To empower them
To reduce need for pain relief
To increase confidence

Most of these statements are sticks, not carrots. The message is either 'It would be good for them', or 'It would be easier for us'. Few if any of these statements are likely to appeal to the women you want to reach. How do you feel about women who do not want to attend classes? Do you find it easy or difficult to stand in their shoes? What insights and information would help you to empathize with their priorities and points of view?

What are the barriers?

There are many different reasons why parents do not attend classes. The times may be unsuitable, the venue may be off-putting or difficult to get to, or the costs of travel may be too great (Cliff and Deery, 1997). Some parents do not come because they are unclear about the benefits (Michie *et al.*, 1990). Others lack confidence and find the idea of joining a group of strangers too daunting.

People tend to avoid situations that they perceive as threatening or alien and in which they fear that they might be judged, stigmatized or isolated (see Maslow's hierarchy of needs in Chapter 3). Women and men who anticipate that factors such as age, educational background, social situation, lifestyle or ethnicity will set them apart from the rest of the group are unlikely to attend.

Anecdotal evidence suggests that some women avoid classes because they smoke, take drugs or intend to bottle-feed, and assume they will be told yet again that they should change. Others lead unpredictable or chaotic lifestyles and find it impossible to commit themselves to specific times and dates. Women who are preoccupied with survival, socially isolated, or worried about housing, racial abuse, domestic violence or getting enough to eat, may have little time and energy for anything else (Schott and Henley, 1991).

Some women prefer to rely on their family for information and support, and find the idea of going to strangers to learn about birth and parenting very strange. Women of conservative cultures and religions may be concerned about having their modesty offended by explicit discussions, pictures or videos. Some may not come in case men are present (Schott and Henley, 1996).

Negative experiences at school may deter some people from going to anything that could be similar (Cliff and Deery, 1997). There are also people whose coping strategy is avoidance or denial. They prefer not to think about what will or could happen, choosing instead to cope at the time. Niven (1992) cites evidence that the best predictor of non-attendance is an 'avoidant' coping strategy.

The name given to antenatal sessions may also contribute to the problem. 'Parentcraft' sounds as if the task is to weave a baby, 'classes' or 'parent education' smack of school, and the word 'group' may be off-putting for some people. A range of titles has been tried around the country with varying success, but it seems that there is no universally attractive name. You and your colleagues need to work out a title that will be most appealing to the people you want to reach.

Reducing the barriers

Like everyone else, parents who are reluctant to come to classes need to feel safe and accepted and to have non-judgmental support and encouragement. Some may never agree to join a group, preferring one-to-one sessions instead. With a little encouragement, others may be willing to attend. Although they are unlikely to want to be defined by their social status, age, ethnicity or lifestyle, they may feel more comfortable with people who are like them and who share their needs and priorities.

Obtaining resources

Organizing special sessions to meet specific needs usually means a radical re-think and reallocation of resources. In a hard-pressed service that requires evidence of effectiveness and quick results, resources rarely match needs. It takes about two years for the grapevine to spread the word to potential customers. Until people start coming because they have heard from their peers that the classes are non-threatening and fun, you will need to set aside precious time for perhaps only a few people. This is only possible with the rock-solid support of those who allocate scarce resources.

Who leads?

The leader is the single most important factor that determines whether a course succeeds or flounders. The need for trust and empathy is paramount. Continuity of leader or leaders is essential. You do not have to share the culture or lifestyle of the participants, or be of a similar age. You just have to be able suspend judgement on those who run their lives in ways very different from your own, and empathize and enjoy being with them.

Clarify the benefits of coming

Many people do not come because they do not think they will benefit (Michie *et al.*, 1990). Learning about birth and parenting in groups may be inconceivable to people who are used to finding out such things from relatives or neighbours. How can you help them get a clear idea of what you offer?

Redesigning your approach

There is a tendency to carry on doing classes as they have always been done in the hope that eventually they will work for everybody. However, doing the same thing and hoping for a different response rarely works. If you want to attract people who have not attended classes up to now, you need a radical rethink. The first and hardest step of all is to throw out your course plan and all your preconceived ideas about what classes are for, what they should include, and how, when and where they should be run. Next you need to plan every detail of time, place, style, approach and content on the carrot principle. This means identifying and eliminating everything that is off-putting to the people you want to reach, focusing on their needs, priorities and concerns, and thinking about what would be appealing and inviting to them. Step into their shoes and consider the following.

Time and place

Where would be most accessible and acceptable, and involve the least possible travel costs? Most people are happier on familiar ground. They may prefer to meet in local community centres or even the upstairs room of a pub rather than on health service premises. However, some may prefer the anonymity of a clinical setting. What time of day would fit in best with other commitments and with their lifestyle? Would your sessions be better attended if they were tacked onto antenatal visits?

Style and approach

What would appeal to the people you want to reach? Whatever their background or circumstances, sessions should be geared to their needs as they see them. Different groups have different needs. However, these common factors are important if you want to attract and keep them coming:

- identifying the benefits to them of coming and using these in all verbal and written invitations
- informality – a relaxed, warm and friendly environment
- refreshments
- identifying and deal with their priorities, even though these may not come within the usual scope of parent education. If they are concerned about housing, or about adapting their wardrobe to cope with expanding waistlines, these are your priorities. This may mean that you cover none of the topics you would normally deal with in an antenatal class

- a flexible, sensitive approach, combined with a willingness to change topics at the drop of a hat
- a client led group, with plenty of opportunities to support and learn from each other
- a flexible programme of rolling classes and drop-in sessions
- free samples or a nearly-new swap shop
- providing information on housing and maternity benefits and local sources of help and support
- organizing a buddy system so that nobody is alone when they walk in for the first time.

Resist the pull to try to change people's behaviour – you might drive them away. It is vital to give wholehearted and genuine praise for any effort, no matter how small, that parents make to improve the health of themselves or their baby.

Setting up support

As we have said, it seems to take about two years for a new venture to become established. It is important to be realistic about this timescale, otherwise it is easy to get disheartened and to give up. Class leaders tend to work in isolation, and those who work with people who do not come to standard classes are often more isolated than the rest. Reaching out to people who are socially excluded can be distressing, so you need and deserve opportunities to let off steam and celebrate your successes. However, it can also be rewarding. One experienced midwife said:

> *It's what I like best because they really need me. The rest can get it somehow – books or friends or whatever – but for these women, it's me or nothing.*

Key points

- Expectant parents represent a cross-section of the population, so antenatal sessions need to cater for a variety of needs.
- Parents with differing needs can either be incorporated into existing classes, be offered one-to-one sessions, or invited to specially designed classes.
- The things that expectant parents have in common more than balance the differences.
- It is essential to examine your own assumptions and preconceived ideas so that you can set them aside.
- The individual is the expert on his or her needs and priorities. Ask tactful and respectful questions.
- Nobody wants to feel marginalized, so include everyone's perspective.
- Confidentiality and respect are paramount.

- Ground rules can be used to ensure that everyone is treated with respect.
- People who avoid classes do so for a variety of reasons.
- Meeting needs may mean throwing out preconceived ideas about what classes are for and when, where and how they should be run, and redesigning them to suit the people you want to encourage.

References

Baker, K. (1999). Young, pregnant ... and pleased. *Practising Midwife*, **2**(3), 14–16.

Braun, D. (1998). And baby makes ... . *New Generation*, Jun, 14–15.

Bryan, A. (2000). The psychosocial effects of infertility and the implications for midwifery practice. *MIDIRS Midwifery Digest*, **10**(1), 8–12.

Carty, E.(1995). Disability, pregnancy and parenting. In: *Aspects of Midwifery Practice, A Research-based Approach* (J. Alexander, V. Levy and S. Roch, eds). Macmillan.

Cliff, D. and Deery, R.(1997). Too much like school: social class, age, marital status and attendance/non-attendance at antenatal classes. *Midwifery*, **13**, 139–45.

Guirdham, M. (1990). *Interpersonal Skills at Work*, p. 31. Prentice Hall.

Kitzinger, C. (1983). Loving women. In: *Woman's Experience of Sex*, p. 106. Penguin Books.

Maternity Alliance (1999). *Maternity Services for Women With Learning Difficulties*. Maternity Alliance.

Michie, S., Marteau, T. M. and Kidd, J. (1990). Antenatal classes: knowingly undersold? *Journal of Reproductive and Infant Psychology*, **3**, 45–53.

Mumford, D. and Bhavsar, U. (1993). Hands-on parentcraft classes for visually impaired people. *Disability, Pregnancy and Parenthood International*, Jan, 6–7.

National Childbirth Trust (1985). *The Emotions and Experiences of some Disabled Mothers*. National Childbirth Trust.

Niven, C. (1992). *Psychological Care for Families: Before, During and After Birth*. Butterworth-Heinemann.

Saffron, L. (1999). Meeting the needs of lesbian clients. *The Practising Midwife*, **2**(11), 18–19.

Sanders, M. (2000). *As Good As Your Word ... A Guide to Community Interpreting and Translation in Public Services*. Maternity Alliance.

Schott, J. and Henley, A. (1991). *Breaking The Barriers. A Training Package on Equal Access to Maternity Services*. Bloomsbury and Islington Health Authority.

Schott, J. and Henley, A. (1996). *Culture, Religion and Childbearing in a Multiracial Society – A Handbook for Health Professionals*. Butterworth-Heinemann.

SHAP (2000). *Calendar of Religious Festivals*. SHAP (see useful addresses).

Singh, D. and Newburn, M. (2000). *Becoming a Father: Men's Access to Information and Support about Pregnancy, Birth and Life with a New Baby*. The National Childbirth Trust.

Wilton, T. (1996). Caring for the lesbian client: homophobia and midwifery. *British Journal of Midwifery*, **14**(3), 126–31.

Wilton, T. (1999). Towards an understanding of the cultural roots of homophobia in order to provide a better midwifery service to lesbian clients. *Midwifery*, **15**, 154–64.

Chapter 18

Shared course leadership

This chapter discusses the advantages and disadvantages of having several people leading a course, and the factors that help leaders to work co-operatively and provide a coherent set of classes that meet parents' needs.

Single or multiple leaders?

Antenatal courses are often led by more than one person. Some are shared equally by two or more people, and some are run by one person who invites others in for particular time slots or topics. Sometimes people from different disciplines lead different parts of a course – for example, a health visitor covers baby care, a midwife deals with labour, and a physiotherapist teaches physical skills. Sometimes each class in a course is led by a different person.

Having different people lead different parts of a course may seem an efficient and flexible way to use staff and ensure that parents meet different members of the team. However, unless there is careful co-ordination, a shared course can have major disadvantages for both parents and class leaders. Often little or no time is allocated for the leaders to get together. Sometimes nobody has overall responsibility for the course, and the content is duplicated or contradictory.

Lack of co-ordination and discontinuous leadership result in a patchwork approach. Leaders may hope that parents will be able build the separate bits into a coherent whole and get what they want. In fact, parents have to keep adjusting to different leaders, styles and approaches. People learn best from those they know and trust. If leaders keep changing, parents may never feel safe enough to ask difficult questions or bring up sensitive issues. It is hard to create or maintain an interactive learning group if the leadership changes frequently, and without group experiences parents never get to know each other and so the social benefits of the course disappear.

This way of running classes also creates problems for leaders. If each is given responsibility for running a small part of the course and is restricted to certain topics, skills or ideas, their ability to react to what happens in the class is very limited. They may feel that they cannot deal with some of the topics that parents bring up, or they may find it hard to change the pace and types of activity in response to unexpected changes of mood or need. With little or no notion of how their contribution fits into the course as a whole, their input can become mechanical or ritualized. They may also lose out on feedback about their portion, or about the course as a whole.

When two or more people share the leadership of a course, leading as a team is likely to be the most effective way to meet parents' needs. Team leadership does not just happen. Like all partnerships, it requires time, thought and commitment. All those involved in leading the course need to think together, plan together and review together. Even if they never work together in a class, the team can still be strong and effective if all its members are equally committed to making the course work, share equal responsibility for what happens, and present themselves to the parents as a co-ordinated unit.

Leading as a team

The benefits

Many people lead courses very successfully on their own, but sharing the leadership has many benefits that amply repay the time and effort involved. In a team, there is someone to think and plan with, someone to bounce ideas off and to learn from, someone to give you constructive feedback, to listen when the going gets tough, and to have fun with! Working as a team eases the isolation that many leaders feel. Your product, whether it is a book like this one or an antenatal course, is likely to be improved as a result of having input from two heads rather than one. Your group, too, will benefit from having two (or more) leaders who offer different styles and role models. This greatly increases the chances of parents finding a style and role model that are right for them. 'Comedians have long known that they can hold their audience for longer when there are two of them' (Bligh, 1998).

Potential blocks

There are also several reasons why it may be difficult to establish and maintain effective leadership teams. It may be hard to find time to work together. People who have always run classes in their own personal way may resist change. Co-operation may be hampered by health professionals guarding certain skills or knowledge and regarding them as their own personal province.

You may have feelings and fears that make you reluctant to lead as a team. Some people feel possessive and do not want to share the work. Others may feel threatened by each other's ideas and skills or are unwilling to share their own, either because they fear they are not good enough or because someone else might steal them. They may feel superior or irritated by some of the things their co-leader does or does not do.

Steps to effective team leadership

You and your co-leaders will only achieve effective team leadership if all of you are willing to offer each other honesty and trust. The larger the number of leaders involved in a course, the more time, tolerance and discussion are needed so that everyone feels included and respected. It may be a slow process.

- Invite your co-leader(s) to spend some time thinking about the way all of you work – or could work – together.
- Arrange a time and place where you can be together without interruption. It may help to agree on confidentiality, and it is important that each of you is careful to take equal time to talk whilst your co-leader(s) listen.
- Depending on how well you and your co-leaders know each other, it may be useful to spend time finding out a bit about each other. This could include something about your life outside work.
- Spend some time listening to each other's aims, philosophy, and approach to leading antenatal classes.
- Listen carefully and respectfully to the differences in approach. These differences can enrich the course rather than cause problems. If necessary, talk them through, now or later, and seek compromise and balance.
- Allocate time for each of you to talk about your own strengths and skills. This can be difficult, as many of us are uncomfortable about what feels like boasting. However, it is important to exchange this information. What do you enjoy doing? Then, what do you find hard or dislike doing?
- Talk about what you like (or think you will like) about working together, and then about what might be hard or could be improved.
- Identify ways in which you could enhance each other's skills and abilities.

End by each of you saying what you have liked or found helpful about examining the way you work together. Plan regular reviews.

You could also draw up an agreement about the way you will work together. One way of doing this is for each of you to write a list of all the qualities and behaviours that you would like from your co-leaders. *These must also be things that you are prepared to offer in return.* The lists can then be shared, clarified and discussed, and used as a basis for reaching consensus on how you will work together. At follow-up meetings, build in time to review what has gone well since you last met and identify areas that need attention.

Having got to know and understand each other better, the next steps are as follows.

Plan together

The only way to ensure that parents receive a comprehensive and coherent package is to plan the course together. The method described in Chapter 16 is a useful tool for joint planning. If disagreements arise, focus on the cards rather than on each other, and keep asking, 'What would work best for parents?'. If you still disagree, review the evidence for the different points of view. If you still cannot reach a consensus you will need find a compromise, or perhaps try out different approaches and then review and decide which works best.

Having agreed a basic core curriculum for your class, try using a course check card for each set of classes (see Chapter 16). This will enable all of you to keep track of what has been covered and what remains to be done.

Start together

If at all possible, start the first class together. This has many advantages. Both or all of you participate in the initial introductions, and, if you are setting ground rules or finding out what the participants want, each of you is then part of the process. People get to know both or all of you at the same time, and are more likely to view you as a team. If you do not start the group together, you will need to decide how to prepare the class for changes of leadership. It is very hard to come into a group that has already been working together and has ideas about what to expect of their leader. Group members may feel apprehensive or resentful of having to adjust. New leaders may also feel anxious about meeting people who already know each other and who may compare them to their colleagues.

The way you prepare the class for a change of leader is important. The participants need to know from the outset that the leadership will be shared. The words you use to tell them are only a small part of the message you convey. If you simply inform them that someone else will lead the next session, they may feel let down or even abandoned. This makes a difficult task even harder for the second leader. If, on the other hand, you set the scene for co-leading right from the start, and speak of your colleague with warmth, as you would speak of one friend to another, the class will be more receptive. Even if you do not particularly warm to your co-leaders, it is important to speak of them with respect.

Work flexibly

How are you going to decide who does what? You do not have to stick to rigid roles, professional boundaries or old ways of working. Everyone can learn to lead effective relaxation sessions (see Chapter 11), just as all leaders can develop the skills needed to start and maintain good group discussion (see Chapter 7). Teamwork can be an opportunity for leaders to develop new skills, with the unusual advantage of having each other to learn from.

As your own repertoire grows, you can vary activities according to the immediate needs and mood of the group rather than sticking to the agreed schedule or preconceived domains. For example, if you had planned to cover the early days of parenting but find that the group is sluggish and unresponsive, you might decide to practise second stage positions instead. Your idea of discussing obstetric interventions may have to be postponed because all the parents can think about is last night's television programme on immunization. A flexible approach allows you to respond immediately to the needs of the group. However, your co-leaders need to be happy with this, and you need to use a course check card or some other method of record keeping that allows everyone to keep track of what has been covered.

Communicate regularly

Telling each other how the class is going, what you covered and what parents are especially interested in is vital. However, if parents tell you something about themselves on a one-to-one basis that you think your co-leader(s) should know, ask the parents' permission before passing the information on.

Model co-operation

Another reason why parents will benefit from effective shared leadership is that you can model co-operation, compromise and tolerance to parents who are in long-term relationships and who are preparing to take on their own joint venture – looking after a baby. They will need to find out each other's views, beliefs and opinions about child rearing, and to identify their own and their partner's strengths and weaknesses. They will have to accept that there is more than one way of doing most things, and work for compromise. Your demonstration of flexibility and respect for each others' skills and points of view will be more effective than anything you can tell them about how they themselves might become a team.

Key points

- When several different people lead different parts of a course, there is a risk that parents' needs will not be met.

- Leading part of a course can also have drawbacks for leaders.
- Leading as a team can reduce problems and help to ensure that parents' needs are met.
- Co-leaders need to spend time getting to know and understand each other.
- Co-leaders need to:
  - plan the course together
  - whenever possible, start the course together
  - work flexibly
  - communicate with each other regularly.

References

Bligh, D. (1998). *What's the Use of Lectures?*, 3rd edn. Intellect.

Chapter 19

Difficult behaviours

Sooner or later, class leaders come across people who behave in ways that are distracting or disruptive. Some may dominate, tell horror stories, behave as if they know it all already, challenge, whisper to their neighbour, or demand endless technical detail and statistics. Others may joke, or make it quite clear with their body language that they would rather be watching TV, down the pub, or anywhere other than in an antenatal class.

Starting with yourself

How do you (or might you) feel when people behave in some of these ways? Class leaders describe a whole range of reactions ranging from irritation, inadequacy, loss of concentration and confidence, to an urge to retaliate, disappear though a hole in the floor or never lead a class again. Unfortunately, people whose behaviour is challenging seem to sense the leader's discomfort and become even more challenging. The result is a potentially escalating cycle of negative actions and reaction. This is detrimental for everyone involved. The trick is to break the cycle and balance the needs of individuals with those of the group as a whole.

Identifying the underlying causes

The most important thing to remember is that *there is a difference between the person and their behaviour*. We know this about ourselves. At times we may be unco-operative, economical with the truth, or respond to certain situations by withdrawing or taking over. However, we know that we do not *always* behave in these ways, and we are highly unlikely to define ourselves by these behaviours. If this is true of us, then it must be true of others. Still, the tendency to confuse a person's behaviour with their personality is common, and is more likely when we think the behaviour is inappropriate or when it affects us adversely (Guirdham, 1990, pp. 64–5). It may be tempting to label people and to assume that the behaviour defines the whole person, but it is unhelpful and leaves us no room for manoeuvre.

There is also a tendency to assume that the problem lies solely with the person who is making life difficult. This is not necessarily the case. Have you ever taken an instant dislike to someone for no apparent reason? On reflection, you may realize that this person (or their behaviour) reminds you of someone with whom you have had problems in the past. It may simply be that they have the same name or tone of voice, or that they look similar. It may be that certain behaviours evoke a particularly strong reaction in you because they are all too familiar. Responding to someone on the basis of your own past experience is unhelpful, so if you find yourself taking an instant dislike to someone or reacting strongly to their behaviour, ask yourself who or what this reminds you of. Then, try to differentiate the past from the present. One way of doing this is to identify all the ways in which this person is different from whoever you had problems with in the past.

Having reflected on your own attitudes and reactions to the situation, the next step is to think about what drives people to behave in these ways. On reflection, many leaders have found that the common denominator is anxiety. This may be due to: a reluctance to come to classes in the first place, embarrassment, fear of feeling a fool, fear of inadequacy, worry about loss of autonomy and control, or concern about fitting in or maintaining status. Each of us has a tendency to react in certain ways to stressful situations. Some people contain their anxiety, while others react in ways that are distracting or disruptive. You will probably find it easier to deal with disruptive or distracting behaviours if you regard them as a person's coping strategy rather than as a deliberate attempt to make your life difficult!

Indirect strategies

Responding directly to the behaviour – for example by challenging it, or responding to aggression with anger or defensiveness – is often futile and tends to increase the tension. The most effective strategy is to tackle the underlying causes (Guirdham, 1990, p. 127). You can allay or reduce some of the fears that people bring to classes by: offering a warm welcome, ensuring physical comfort, helping everyone to feel part of the group, demonstrating respect, and eliciting and following their agenda (see Chapter 5).

Small group work

You can interrupt most unhelpful behaviours by frequent use of small group work. However, make sure that the person who is being disruptive is not always in the same group! When you work with the whole group it is easier for people to dominate, challenge, joke and even heckle. You are also much more likely to be distracted and disheartened by people's negative body language or whispering.

Small group work removes you from the limelight and gives you time to regain your composure. It can give you time to listen, one-to-one, to the person who is dominating or telling horror stories, and if necessary fix a time to listen after the class. It is also ideal for quiet people who do not want to speak in the large group.

The group's agenda

Use the group's agenda as a reason to move on. Make a polite but firm statement, such as 'I'm going to stop you there as time is short and there is still a lot that you asked to cover'. You can add emphasis by drawing the group's attention to the list of topics that they asked for (see Chapter 5). This is likely to enlist co-operation from the majority, as it demonstrates that your intention is to deal with what they want.

Direct strategies

If the person does not respond to indirect approaches, you may need to be more direct. It is best to choose a way that neither puts the person down nor involves you in an argument; otherwise you will lose the trust of the group even if you 'win' that particular encounter.

Try not to get into the situation where you are coping with someone's unhelpful behaviour whilst the group sits back and watches the struggle. If you find it a problem the rest of the group does too, so they have just as much interest in resolving it as you do. If you can deal with such difficulties as being a problem *for the group* and not just for you, the better the outcome of any intervention is likely to be.

The following examples give some tips for dealing with some common behaviours.

People who tell horror stories

People who tell horror stories or dwell on one particular topic need to let off steam, and trying to stop them seldom works. You can set aside time for them do this with the full attention of the group. The speaker must know how long he or she has (say a maximum of five minutes), and that they will not be interrupted. This may be all that is needed, but should anyone continue longer than their allotted time, try saying firmly and politely, 'I'm going to stop you there', and then offer time after the class instead.

People who are quiet

Leaders usually feel better if everyone is contributing, but some parents feel worse if they are under pressure to speak, especially in a large group. The fact that some people do not talk freely does not necessarily mean that they are not benefiting from the class. Small groups will usually provide enough safety for quieter people to talk if they want to.

People who joke

Jokes can be entertaining, but they are also a way of dealing with sensitive and embarrassing issues and of exerting control. The occasional quip lightens the atmosphere, but jokes that trivialize or exaggerate issues need to be balanced with reality – 'well it might sound a bit like popping a cork out of a bottle, but the second stage takes much longer and is usually very hard work for the mother. Let's think about how it might feel and what you can do'.

If people persist in joking, try asking questions that acknowledge the real feelings and fears behind the jokes – 'How do you think you might really feel if that happened?' – or ask them to hold back – 'We can come back to that later, but let's start by covering the things that are more likely to happen'.

Sexual innuendo and jokes that demean people are harder to handle. It is usually better to speak to the person individually, either during small group work or after the class. You could try asking how he or she feels about coming to classes, and what issues that particular person wants to cover. Then explain the consequences on the class of their joking ('some people find it distasteful'; 'there is no way we can get through everything if you constantly distract us') and ask them to stop.

People who never listen

If you have established rules about listening with respect to each other, you can remind people to abide by them. If not, you could point out that things will get missed if people talk at the same time, and suggest that they speak one at a time. Don't allow interruptions – 'Hang on Michelle, can you just wait until Lorraine has finished?'.

People who want detailed information

Some people deal with anxiety by amassing information. Niven (1992) uses the term 'vigilant' to describe people who seek out statistics and detailed information about everything that could possibly happen. The needs of vigilant people have to be balanced with the needs of everyone else in the group. If requests for more and more detail and statistics are beginning to dominate the class, you can offer to deal with these on an individual basis. Another strategy is to shift the focus from acquiring information to using it (see Chapters 7–9 for small group work ideas).

People with fixed ideas

Strongly held views are never relinquished easily, and some people think that changing one's mind is a sign of weakness. Direct challenges to people's beliefs usually fail. A relaxed approach combined with some of the indirect strategies described above is likely to be the best approach.

Occasionally you may be able to help someone take a more balanced view (see 'Adjusting information' in Chapter 9), but it is unrealistic to expect to change someone else's views.

In conclusion

If you are lucky the group will deal with the situation for you; however, you also need to ensure that the person is not picked on. Occasionally, despite all your best endeavours, you may be unable to reduce disruptive behaviours. We have found that the best way to cope is to put it down to experience and visualize ourselves having a much more positive and rewarding experience with the next group we lead.

Key points

- The cycle of escalating anxiety that inappropriate behaviour can trigger affects everyone adversely and needs to be broken.
- There is a difference between the person and their behaviour. Labelling or defining a person on the basis of one aspect of their behaviour is unhelpful.
- The underlying cause of difficult and inappropriate behaviour is nearly always anxiety.
- Dealing with underlying causes usually works better than tackling the overt behaviour.
- Indirect strategies often work well.
- Use specific strategies with care so that anxiety is decreased rather than increased.
- You may not always succeed!

References

Guirdham, M. (1990). *Interpersonal Skills at Work*. Prentice Hall.
Niven, C. (1992). *Psychological Care for Families: Before, During and After Birth*. Butterworth-Heinemann.

Chapter 20

Evaluating your classes

This chapter discusses the importance of evaluation, and describes ways in which you can assess your effectiveness.

Why evaluate?

There are both personal and organizational reasons for evaluating classes:

- You need to know how you are doing in order to remain effective and develop your personal and professional skills.
- Managers who have to find the resources for classes may want to monitor attendance rates and ensure that the standard of all the classes in their area is good.

Measuring effectiveness

Assessing the effectiveness of parent education is not easy. A whole range of factors may influence outcomes, including, for example, the aspirations and lifestyles of the parents who attend; the length and content of the course; the leader's style, approach and skills; and the degree to which the clinical care that parents receive reflects and relates to the content and philosophy of the classes they attend.

Objective data are desirable in a culture that demands facts and figures to justify providing services, but such data may not reflect the quality of classes, nor ensure that parents' needs are met. Measures of effectiveness that are drawn up unilaterally and without consulting parents are more likely to indicate the agendas and assumptions of the class leader and the organization in which she works than the needs and priorities of parents. For example:

- outcomes such as breastfeeding rates are more likely to be a measure of decisions that women made long before coming to classes, of the amount of help, support or conflicting advice they receive, of whether they themselves were breastfed, and of the attitude of her partner and peers (OPCS, 1992).

- attendance levels may simply reflect the socio-economic status of the women in the area.
- assessing the use of analgesia in labour conflicts with the principle of informed choice, since the decision to have an epidural is as legitimate as the decision to decline one. Anyway, labour ward protocols and the attitudes of labour ward staff are likely to be a far more powerful influence on what happens during labour than any antenatal class (Nolan, 1994; Leeseberg Stamler, 1998).

Although some objective measures can be useful, the subjective responses of parents are also important. If parents seek out classes, find them informative and supportive, and as a result become more confident and able to take responsibility for themselves and their baby, then the classes have served a useful purpose (Shearer, 1993).

In practice, the benefits to parents and their children of antenatal classes may only emerge weeks, months or even years later, and so may not be apparent to the people who teach or manage them. For example, parents have helped their children to manage pain by teaching them relaxation and breathing techniques. They have used massage to help teenagers stressed by exams. They have learned to deal with stressful situations by taking one thing at a time. 'Learning is best conceived as a process, not in terms of outcomes' (Kolb, 1984).

Evaluating your performance

So how can you find out about your classes? You can gain a certain amount of information by collecting and analysing numbers. How many women come to your class compared with the total number giving birth in the catchment area? Seeing this proportion rise would be one sign of success. How many come because of word-of-mouth recommendation? See how many people complete the whole course. Of course some women may have their babies early, but if many people attend erratically or drop out after a few classes, it may be time for a re-think.

You could also count how many people want to come and can't get a place. Is the number rising? If demand far outstrips your ability to meet it, this may bring its own stresses, but it also satisfying to know that you are offering what people want.

Self-assessment

Reflection is an important part of ongoing personal and professional development. Many class leaders quietly assess themselves most of the time.

At the end of each class, try asking yourself the questions listed below. You will notice that the questions start by looking at a positive. If you know what you do well, you can repeat and build on it. If you concentrate on what went badly, it is easy to feel despondent and hopeless. We suggest that, as a rough rule of thumb, 80 per cent of the time should be spent looking at what you do well, and 20 per cent looking at what you could improve and how. Whichever method you use to assess your skills, you will benefit most if you stick to the 80 : 20 ratio.

- *What did I do well?* Nothing is too trivial! Acknowledging and integrating a late arrival, remembering people's names, noticing that some people need further explanations of some aspect of labour, leading the relaxation at a slow gentle pace, ending the class on a warm note – these are all signs of your skill as a leader. Acknowledge them.
- *How do I know?* Think about the effects of your actions – what signs were there that what you did was helpful? For example, 'I know that taking a minute to welcome Kate helped, because she settled in and became part of the group straight away'; or 'I know that my explaining X in more detail helped because David said he found it clear and there was a look of understanding on other people's faces'.
- *What could I improve and how?* Resist the temptation to answer this until you have extracted all the positive thoughts from the event. Identify one or two areas that you want to improve, and choose a priority. This should be something that you think you can achieve reasonably soon and without too much difficulty, and something that would improve the quality of your classes. For example, if you are new to leading classes and tend to rely heavily on giving information, your first step could be to introduce some group work, a discussion or an activity.

Decide precisely what do you want to achieve, then consider questions like:

- where or from whom could I get input or help?
- what steps do I need to take to set this up?
- when will I take the first step?
- when will I review?

Getting feedback from parents

We believe that parents are the most important source of information on the quality and effectiveness of antenatal classes. There is a range of ways, both formal and informal, of finding out what parents think about your classes. We suggest you use a variety of approaches.

Informal approaches

You can use these throughout the course. They have the advantage of giving you time to respond and adjust what you are doing. If you only hear from parents at the end of the course, it is too late to change. Informal approaches include:

- observing the way group members interact and respond to what you are doing
- establishing their agenda and asking them to tell you when an item has been covered sufficiently – 'Is it too simple to ask parents at the outset what they want, and then ask them afterward if they got it?' (Shearer, 1993)
- leading a round at the end of the class and inviting each person to tell you something they found particularly interesting or useful (see Chapter 5 for how to do a round). People often notice and appreciate things that you are not even aware of or did not think particularly significant. You could do a similar exercise at the end of the whole course
- asking at the beginning of a class, 'Have you been thinking about anything particular since the last class? Is there anything you want to know more about?'

Formal approaches

You can also do a more formal review by asking parents to fill in an evaluation form. The feedback you get will vary depending on what you ask and when you ask for it. Will it be at the end of the last class of the course? After the course is finished? Immediately after, or a few weeks or months after the babies are born?

Waiting makes things more complicated because it involves mailing questionnaires and you are unlikely to get a good response. However, you may decide that it is worth taking the trouble, since asking for feedback when some time has elapsed gives a clearer view of the real impact of your course. An alternative is to hold a reunion and use part of the time for feedback (see below). This also allows parents to begin debriefing, and can give you an opportunity to spot people who, because of their experiences, may need more support.

If you ask for written evaluation, you need to decide what kind of form you will use. A structured form that invites only Yes/No answers is easy for most people to fill in and straightforward to collate, but offers limited information. You will get richer responses if you use headings to focus people's thinking on various aspects of the class, and leave them plenty of space for their responses. However, people who are unused to expressing themselves on paper are unlikely to write much or enjoy the experience. A compromise is to combine the two approaches in a form that contains predominantly closed questions with a few open ones at the end such as:

- what did you enjoy most about the classes?
- what did you find most useful?
- what did you wish we had included or spent more time on?
- what improvements can you suggest?

You could also include a scale and ask people to indicate how useful they found the classes by circling a number between one and ten – one being not at all useful, ten being extremely useful.

It is enlightening if everyone in the locality uses the same evaluation form. You may want to get together with other class leaders to review existing forms and devise one that everyone can use.

Using the reunion

An excellent time for getting feedback is at a class reunion. This is usually timed for a few weeks after the last baby in the group is due. Although participants will probably have their hands too full of babies to fill in forms, you can structure the session so that each person has an opportunity to tell the group about the birth and her or his experience of early parenthood. If you have a large class you may need to divide them up into small groups so that they all have time to tell their stories and be listened to. You can then ask each person questions like the open ones mentioned above.

Accepting feedback from parents

If you ask for feedback you must be prepared to accept *all* the responses you get. Sometimes participants who appeared to enjoy the classes hugely, and to gain support and confidence from them, say afterwards that they didn't help much. Or someone will say about a topic you covered thoroughly 'You never told us about X'. Sometimes the others say, 'Oh yes, she did'. Whatever the response, you need to accept the criticism or comment cheerfully, or you may get no more feedback from this group! Many parents focus on the positive in order to avoid hurting the leader's feelings, so you may need to encourage them to suggest improvements as well. Telling them that their comments play an important part in helping you to ensure that your classes continue to be useful to parents may elicit helpful feedback.

Long-term review

Every few months, take an overall look at your teaching. This will be more effective if you have someone to assist you and to take some notes for you to keep.

Your assistant's role is to listen, to keep you going, and to remind you to be detailed and specific. They can ensure that you stick to the ratio of 80 per cent successes to 20 per cent improvements, and encourage you to celebrate your skills and abilities and to believe that you can develop still further. One way your assistant can help is to ask a series of questions and then listen carefully to the answers, jotting down any useful information that arises. For example:

- What are you doing well in your classes? Be very specific and detailed, and give examples of the effects of each skill you identify. Nothing is too trivial.
- Outline any changes and improvements you have made to your course. If you set goals at your last review, take time to appreciate what you achieved.
- If you did not reach a previous goal, identify why. What have you found hard?
- What would you like to improve? What input or resources do you need? How will you set about arranging to get these?
- What input or ongoing training have you had since your last review?

In the next 6 months/year:

- How do you see your classes changing or developing? For example, are there any organizational changes in the pipeline?
- What changes do you personally want to make to your classes? How exactly will you set about achieving these?
- What is your order of priority for these?
- What input or support do you need? Where and when could you get it?
- What is your first step?
- End by setting a date for your next review.

Peer assessment

Another way of finding out how you are doing is to invite a colleague or interested friend to sit in on your class, possibly just once, or through a whole course. This may sound pretty daunting! Many people's memories of assessment, performance appraisal and feedback provoke winces rather than smiles. However, it does not have to be that way. If you use the 80 : 20 ratio you will find out what you do well, which is good for confidence, and focusing on what you want to improve and how you will achieve it gives you a constructive way forward.

Think carefully about whom you choose. Find someone you trust and respect and who will be constructive, open and honest. Most of us have feelings of competitiveness or not being good enough. These feelings can be recognized, discussed and set aside, but if either of you holds them strongly in relation to the other, pairing up will probably not be fruitful.

Your observer might start by reading through this chapter. Then you will need to do some careful preparation together.

Preparation

You need to agree what your observer will be looking for. She might observe the class as a whole, noting specifically what went well. People with less experience as observers may find it easier to concentrate on one or two specific aspects of each class. Here are some examples of areas to focus on.

- Your skills as a group leader – is everyone included and involved?
- The atmosphere – is it relaxing and welcoming?
- Your appearance – dress, tone of voice and body language.
- Your language – is it inclusive and jargon free? Can you convey technical information clearly and simply?
- Discussion – is it usually channelled through you, or do participants talk to each other?
- Pace – are participants interested and actively involved throughout the class?
- Your skill in teaching relaxation, positions or massage.
- Your ability to respond flexibly to questions and issues that arise spontaneously.
- Your skills in welcoming and involving partners and meeting their needs.
- Your inclusion of the baby as a sensitive individual.

Other issues also need sorting out before the class. Where will the observer sit? If she is straight opposite you, you will be constantly reminded of her presence and tempted to focus on her. If she is out of your sight, you may worry about her reactions. What will her role in the group be? Will she sit silently? Will she contribute when she wants, or wait for you to invite her comments? What about taking notes, bearing in mind that other people find it uncomfortable or distracting to have someone writing things down?

Preparing the participants

When someone new joins a group, the dynamics change. You have only to think what it's like when you begin to relax at a party, thinking all the guests are present, only to have the doorbell ring and be required to adjust to someone new. Participants will need forewarning that someone else will be joining the class. Tell them why the assessor is coming, otherwise they might wonder who is being observed! When she arrives, introduce her, remind the group of her role, and perhaps do a round of names.

Reviewing the class

Whenever possible, arrange to talk about the class straight afterwards. It will then be fresh in your minds, and you are spared the trauma of waiting.

Receiving feedback

When you are offered feedback, the most important thing is to listen and accept what you hear. This is easier said than done. Curiously, it is usually particularly hard to listen to what went well, so you may have to make a real effort to take in what is being said. If you find it hard to believe positive feedback, or are unclear about precisely what you did well, ask for more detail. This is not selfish, bigheaded or boastful. Once you know, you can repeat good practice and grow in confidence.

Keep on listening when improvements are suggested. If you think these are valid, review with your observer the various ways in which you could achieve them. If you don't think a suggestion is valid, ask for more detail about what has been said. If you still find it hard to accept, check it out with someone else who you trust to be honest with you. If you then see the relevance, look for ways of improving. If you decide that the observation is not valid, set it aside with the proviso that you might review it in the future, especially if someone else makes the same observation.

Giving feedback

Giving feedback is only useful if it helps the person you are giving it to. Constructive feedback focuses mainly on the positive, and is most effective when it is detailed and specific. Giving facts is nearly always useful, whereas your personal views and opinions are unlikely to help the other person. If you can substantiate your comments with examples of the effects of the person's skills or actions, she is more likely to absorb what you are telling her.

It helps to focus on what the leader did rather than on her personality or attitudes. The former is easier to hear and act on. When you are giving feedback about what might be improved, keep it to a minimum. Nitpicking is not helpful, so stick to the most important factors and only comment on things that she can actually change. For example, you may think smaller classes would benefit the participants, but the leader's manager may be adamant that it is better to have large classes than to exclude people.

If you suggest improvements, assist the person to think about how she might set about achieving them. If you suggest more than one improvement, help her to establish priorities so that the task feels manageable. In all that you say, assume that the person who is receiving your feedback has been doing the best she can at present and that, with support, she can to develop and improve her skills.

Key points

- Evaluation is part of personal and professional development, [illegible] benefits for the organization in which the leader works.
- Objective measures do not necessarily reflect the quality of the classes.
- Parents' views and reactions are a useful guide to what is good and what could be improved.
- It is more effective to use several ways of getting feedback from parents.
- Self and peer assessment are useful tools for assessing and improving skills.
- Focusing on successes for 80 per cent of the time and improvements for 20 per cent of the time helps people to identify and build on what they do well.

References

Kolb, D. A. (1984). *Experiential Learning: Experience as the Source of Learning and Development*. Prentice Hall.

Leeseberg Stamler, L. (1998). The participants' view of childbirth education: is there congruency with an ennoblement framework for patient education? *Journal of Advanced Nursing*, **28**(5), 939–47.

Nolan, M. (1994). Effectiveness of antenatal education. *British Journal of Midwifery*, **2**(11), 534–48.

OPCS (1992). *Infant Feeding*. Office of Population Censuses and Surveys, Social Services Division. HMSO.

Shearer, H. (1993). Commentary: effects of prenatal classes cannot be measured by obstetric management. *BIRTH*, **September**, 130–1.

Chapter 21

Professional development and support

This chapter discusses the needs of the class leader, and outlines ways in which you can plan for your own personal and professional development.

In good antenatal classes parents change, learn, enjoy themselves and benefit in a host of other ways. It is of course rewarding to whoever runs the class to watch these things happen. However, they don't come for free – you give your time, attention and energy in order to meet parents' needs. If you are to remain effective you too need opportunities to learn and to develop your skills, and from time to time you will need support.

Professional development

Whether you are inexperienced, or an old hand at leading classes, you will benefit from regular review (see Chapter 20, training and input). There are a variety of ways in which you can increase your knowledge and improve your skills, and some of these are described below.

Workshops and seminars

Try anything that will enhance and broaden your knowledge and skills. Look out for workshops and training sessions on the process of teaching and communicating, relaxation, exercise, active birth or massage. You could also attend courses on topics such as assertiveness, adult learning, groups and group work, listening skills, counselling techniques or bereavement counselling.

Build networks with others in the field

Each profession or group involved with expectant and young parents has a different perspective on what parents need. For example, midwives have plenty of experience of the issues parents face during pregnancy and labour and the transition to parenthood. Health visitors have much longer contact with parents after the birth, while physiotherapists see women who need treatment during pregnancy and after. Active Birth teachers and National Childbirth Trust teachers, breastfeeding counsellors and people running parent support groups may offer yet another set of insights. Talking to other people who are involved with parents and babies may help you to identify topics and issues that should or could be covered in classes.

Observing antenatal classes

Sitting in on someone else's class can be extremely useful. If you can find time, observe a whole course. If you find someone who is happy for you to come to her classes, the two of you will need to decide exactly what your role will be and how the participants will be prepared for your arrival (see Chapter 20).

Books, leaflets and magazines

There is a steady flood of books and magazines aimed at expectant parents, and a smaller output aimed at their carers. Much of the content is repetitive and some of it may be a passing fashion, but you need to know what parents are reading and keep an eye on what is new. Read articles and reviews in professional journals, and take time for an occasional browse through the books and magazines on pregnancy and parenthood at your local store or newsagent. Check out the publications' lists of voluntary organizations such as the National Childbirth Trust and Maternity Alliance (see 'Useful addresses' at the end of this book).

Surfing the net

There is a huge and growing amount of information on the World Wide Web aimed at expectant and new parents, and there are also websites for health professionals. The quality of the information varies, but it is useful to know what parents might be reading and what other health professionals are thinking.

Using new ideas

When you are inspired by a new approach you may feel that you can't wait to try it; that you have got to go back to square one and change everything, or that, however much you want to, you just cannot see yourself using it. All these reactions are common; however, they need some thought and moderation. Whether you are unsure of yourself or eager to try out something new, you are likely to be more effective if you take one step at a time. So, before you include anything new in your classes or reject a tempting innovation, think about the following.

- Clarify your purpose in including this topic, exercise or approach. How might parents benefit? What do you aim to achieve?
- Examine your own feelings and attitudes to it.
- Explore ways in which others have handled it.

If you decide to try something out:

- Adapt what you have seen so that you use words and approaches that are your own.
- Try it out yourself. Use a tape recorder or a mirror, or practise with a friend or colleague who can give you constructive feedback.
- Fit it into your course plan, linking it to other topics or using it as and when you judge it will be most useful for the group.
- Evaluate by observing the immediate effects and inviting feedback from parents.
- Assess usefulness by listening to parents' reflections after the birth.

Developing your own ideas

A few people seem to have an infinite ability to pull imaginative ideas out of their hats. A much larger number feel unable to innovate or incorporate new ideas. In reality, we all have a greater capacity than we realize to think creatively. Given the right circumstances, we can all adapt existing ideas and build on them. One vital element is the will and energy to have a go.

Ideas tend to come unexpectedly – in the supermarket queue, first thing after waking, in the middle of leading a class, or when you are doing something completely different. Because they come at inconvenient times and are probably incomplete, they get undervalued or ignored. Notice when and where ideas tend to occur to you and, instead of letting them slip away, jot them down, however unworkable or inconvenient they seem.

Later, take time to play with them, exploring even the ones that appear ridiculous or impractical. Then develop your best ideas before you try them out. This process will work much better if you have an interested and attentive listener. You don't have to come up with complete ideas; this is an opportunity to think out loud, to explore and develop your ideas with assistance.

Setting up support

Everyone needs input and support. Leading classes can be rewarding and exciting, but it can also be stressful and difficult. If you have a good support system you can solve problems, let off steam, renew your enthusiasm, and exchange ideas and strategies.

You may be lucky and have support for your clinical role, but your need for support as a class leader may get sidelined by clinical dilemmas and problems. Unless you have time to focus exclusively on leading classes, your own needs are unlikely to be met. You can organize support by setting up your own personal network and by attending meetings for class leaders in your locality. Having more than one forum ensures that you have access to different kinds of input, and that support is always available.

Setting up personal networks

If you have your own support network, you can usually access support whenever you need it. Find two or three people, either colleagues or friends, who would be willing to exchange support either on the telephone or face to face. They do not necessarily have to be class leaders or even health professionals; they just need to be interested in giving and receiving support.

Leaders' meetings

The best ones meet regularly and are large enough to bring together different ideas, yet small enough to allow people to get to know each other. You can use your meetings to share skills and ideas; report back on relevant training, books and articles; let off steam; review a specific topic; or discuss particular issues or difficulties. Every now and then you could work in pairs to do self-assessments (see Chapter 20). You will, however, need to keep the focus on classes and avoid the tendency to revert to discussing your clinical work.

Forming agreements

Successful support depends on people making a commitment to each other and taking time to think about how they will work together. If you set up a personal support network or a class leaders' group, you might find it useful to consider the following.

- *Use of time*. Where will you meet and how often? What time of day is best, and how long will you spend together? If you agree to be available to each other on the telephone, discuss when you would prefer not to be called (e.g. 'Not after nine', or 'Avoid weekends').
- *Confidentiality*. This is often ignored when it comes to colleagues and friends. However, it is vital if you are to feel able to express yourself fully and freely. Each person needs to be certain that nothing they say will be repeated to anyone else.

- *Privacy*. You need a room where you will not be overheard, overlooked or disturbed by people, telephones or personal pagers. In most workplaces this is hard to find, but it is worth making an effort to ensure privacy.
- *Equal time*. Ensure that the time available is divided so that each person has an equal amount of time to talk. This division of time may seem artificial at first, but if you are not scrupulous about it, sooner or later one person will take more than the other(s). Of course there will be times when one person has a crisis or special difficulties and things get out of balance, but everyone deserves a fair share of this valuable asset.
- *Respect*. All participants deserve complete respect because they are doing the very best they can, given their current knowledge and circumstances. Appreciation and respect enhances people's ability to clarify ideas and think creatively. So for example, even if you are listening to ideas that you think are ill conceived, it is important to maintain an attitude of non-judgmental respect *for the person* you are listening to. Respect also includes sticking to arrangements you make to meet or call each other, unless there are exceptional circumstances. If you telephone unexpectedly, check that it is convenient and, if not, fix another time to talk. It is not helpful for either of you to try to talk and listen when the other is distracted by different demands.
- *Competitiveness*. Feelings of competitiveness may creep in, and can spoil relationships if they are not dealt with. Usually competitiveness arises when people do not feel good about themselves, so reminding each other of the qualities and skills each of you has can help. You may also need to come to an agreement about using or adapting each other's ideas. Who do ideas belong to? How can they be used for the benefits of the parents, a goal you hold in common?
- *Trust*. Mutually trusting relationships are to be cherished. Clarify what trust means to each of you so that it can grow and strengthen as you work together.
- *Managing strong feelings*. There may be occasions when someone needs to deal with her feelings before she can think clearly. If someone is angry, frustrated, sad or scared, she may need to let off steam. You can help by having a relaxed, supportive and encouraging approach to someone who needs to express anger or who simply needs to cry.
- *Regular review*. Take time every now and then to review the way your network or group is working. Discuss what is going well, and what could be improved and how. By doing this you can ensure that time is well spent and everyone's needs are met, and you can adapt to emerging needs and changing circumstances.
- *Supportive listening*. One of the most useful things you can offer each other is listening. Having time to think out loud can be liberating and enlightening. As a listener, you do not need to find solutions, give answers, advice or reassurance. *With your attention and approval, the speaker will usually solve her own problems, develop her own thinking and*

reach her own conclusions. Good listening means setting aside your own ideas and thoughts and instead focusing entirely on what the speaker is saying and doing. This is easier said than done, because stray thoughts creep in along with the urge to give advice or tell them what you think. Whenever this happens, resist the temptation to intervene and firmly set your own thoughts aside. With practice, you will find that it gets easier to keep your total attention on the speaker. Resist the temptation to ask questions. Questions should be used sparingly and be carefully thought out. They should only be asked for the benefit of the speaker, and not because you, the listener, would like to know more.

Key points

- Regular input and training are essential for maintaining and developing skills.
- It is important to plan how you will introduce new ideas and approaches.
- Everyone needs and deserves input and support.
- Personal support networks and leaders' groups are more successful when the people involved agree how they will work together.

Chapter 22

Initiating change

This chapter outlines the factors that can help initiate change. As a class leader you may want to initiate change not only in your own approach to leading antenatal classes, but also in the way that classes are set up and run in your locality. You might also want to ensure that the things that parents learn in classes are backed up and supported during and after labour.

Initiating change

Change is seldom easy, especially if you do it from within a hierarchy. Changes that involve and affect other people are the most difficult. Nobody likes being told that they should change, and resistance is a common response, especially when a change is imposed. However, giving up before you start guarantees that nothing will change! There are several ways in which you can make change more likely.

- *Choose one issue*. Start by identifying one issue – not necessarily the most fundamental, but the one you think is most likely to be successful.
- *Gather and evaluate the evidence* for and against the change.
- *Consider your timing*. Every now and again there are times when change and review are easier to initiate because change is already happening – when a unit moves to a new location or two units merge, when protocols are reviewed, or when training or orientation programmes are revised. However, some of these may not necessarily be the best times for you to add new issues. If changes are already causing large amounts of stress, anxiety or extra work either for staff or managers, then one more may be the last straw and you may be more successful if you bide your time.
- *Sound people out*. Assess the level of support, listen to other people's views and adapt your ideas accordingly.
- *Involve the relevant people* in the process. It may seem important to approach someone in a position of authority who might have a direct

and rapid influence on how things are done. However, this may not be appropriate, and is certainly not essential as a first step. You will be more successful if you start by involving people who will be directly affected by the proposed change. If you do not, you are likely to encounter high levels of resistance when they eventually hear about your proposals (Plant, 1987, p. 19).

- *Seek support*. It is never easy to change things alone. You are far less likely to get discouraged and are more likely to succeed in at least raising awareness of issues, if not precipitating actual change, if you do it with input and support from at least one other person.
- *Review current practice*. Raising issues and writing a protocol for a review can lay the foundations for change and can sometimes be enough to precipitate change (Ogden, 2001).
- *Identify the benefits* that the proposed change could bring, not just for parents but for staff as well. If people can see advantages in making a change, they are less likely to resist and more likely to co-operate (Guirdham, 1990).
- *Identify and manage potential blocks and resistance*. According to Plant (1987, p. 29), resistance to change is a natural phenomenon. It is an emotional reaction, and cannot therefore be reduced with logical argument. An important part of managing change is listening to people. This helps people to feel involved, and enables you to identify potential problems and discover what needs to be done to reduce resistance.
- *Use tact and diplomacy*. Being asked to change is stressful, and can make people feel vulnerable. Some colleagues may feel threatened or think that you are implying that what they have been doing all these years is not good enough. Others lack the confidence and the skills to make changes, and need support and input. Be patient; evolution may be slow, but it can also be more successful than revolution.
- *Offer information, skills and support*. People can only change if they have the appropriate skills and information. You may not be in a position to offer these yourself, but you can at least identify people's needs and find ways of meeting them.
- *Review regularly*. When you have identified the issue, sounded people out, gathered some support, and marshalled the evidence or written a proposal for change, take time to review. It may be that by merely raising the issue and encouraging people to think afresh, things have started to change and nothing more needs to be done. Or you may conclude that the resistance will be too great and that the time is not ripe for taking things further.

Here are some examples of how you might apply these principles to specific situations.

Changing the way classes are organized and led

You may want to change several things about the way classes are organized and led in your area. However, you will achieve more if you start with just one. The first step is to gather evidence. Depending on the issue, your sources could include class attendance rates, feedback from parents, surveys, reports from other units who run successful antenatal classes, and a literature search.

Example 1

Let's assume that you think classes should be more parent-centred and interactive. You could start by sounding a few people out and perhaps finding one or two people who agree with you.

You could then invite everyone involved in leading classes to a meeting. Make sure that you include people who may only lead a small part of the course. Choose a time and place that will suit as many people as possible, and provide tea and coffee! You could then outline why you think a change to more interaction and involvement would benefit parents (they would be more relaxed and involved, be more likely to get what they want from classes, and more able make friends), and why the change would benefit leaders (it's more stimulating, fun and rewarding when parents are involved, and the leader does not have to be the sole focus of attention).

You could then demonstrate a way of achieving more involvement, for example by leading your colleagues in an ice-melting process and eliciting an agenda (e.g. for future class leader meetings). This offers them an opportunity to *experience* a method of turning an audience into an interactive group and eliciting an agenda. Afterwards, *ask your colleagues what they think* of the process. This approach offers people the information they need to use the techniques themselves, and a chance to experience them. It also involves people in deciding how to change things.

If some of you decide to initiate the change, make sure that you are available to support each other and that you review the effects of the change. If, as a result of your changes, the classes become more lively and the feedback becomes more positive, you can celebrate your success. If some or all of you have been less than successful, you can discuss the possible reasons and plan for improvements. The few people who are highly resistant to making the change *might* just decide to do so if others are enthusiastic about it.

Example 2

Alternatively you may want to change the structure of the course, so that instead of parents spending one hour on physical skills with one leader and another on information with a second leader, topics, physical skills and discussion are integrated into one two-hour session, perhaps with shared leadership (see Chapter 18).

You could start by assessing the numbers attending classes. What is the drop-out rate? Do some people attend only part of the class? What about the feedback from parents? You could gather evidence for the advantages of frequent changes of pace and activity throughout a class. You could talk to class leaders who use a more integrated approach, and gather evidence for the benefits to parents and class leaders (for example, more variety and frequent changes of pace make it is easier to maintain attention and enthusiasm, people are less likely to be put off different aspects of the class if they only last a short time, it is easier to link topics with skills and coping strategies, and leaders can learn new skills from each other).

You also need to be realistic and identify the potential adjustments that class leaders will have to make. For example, some leaders may have to reorganize their working patterns and clinical commitments in order to fit in with a different way of working. They may have to adjust to a co-operative rather than a solo approach to leadership.

You could then invite the leaders concerned to join you, and outline your reasons and evidence for considering a change. You could try laying out an alternative course plan together. This gives everyone an objective overview of the different ways in which a course can be organized (see Chapter 16). Make sure that you keep your focus on the cards, not on each other. You could also discuss how you could increase co-operation and share the leadership in order to offer a better course to the parents (see Chapter 18). Two (or three) of you might decide also to set up an integrated course as a pilot project and evaluate the pros and cons for parents and for class leaders.

If you encounter resistance, let people talk about why they do not like the idea and why they think it would not work. This may give you insights into what needs to be done to improve the chances of co-operation. Alternatively, it may be prudent to wait and meet again sometime in the future, when everyone has had time to cool down and reflect.

If any of your colleagues decide to make changes, set up a time for everyone to meet again to review how things went, celebrate successes and iron out any difficulties.

Changing patterns of care

The feedback that class leaders get from parents after the birth often includes the parents' perception of the care they received during and after labour. While many parents are appreciative and grateful, some are unhappy about certain aspects of care, and there may be times when the same issue is raised by a series of different parents.

When this happens, the first step is to reflect on what you are saying in classes. Are you offering balanced, objective and realistic information about the issue? Are most parents' expectations realistic? If, after reflection, your answer to these questions is 'no', you need to change your classes. However, if your answer is 'yes', you may conclude that certain aspects of clinical care could be improved and you might decide to do something about it.

If you decide to take action, start by checking that you have heard the same concern from a number of people from different classes. You might ask other class leaders if they have heard the same thing from people in their classes.

For example, over a period of time you may hear from many different women that they did not get as much help as they had expected with relaxation and breathing, or that they were discouraged from moving about freely during labour. Or a significant number of parents may say that they were unhappy that their partner was asked to leave soon after the birth. Alternatively, you may hear about an increasing number of women undergoing artificial rupture of membranes, or receiving conflicting advice about breastfeeding. Parents might tell you that nobody showed them how to bath their baby, or those who decide to bottle-feed may say that nobody showed them how to prepare feeds.

Once you have chosen your issue, start discussing it with colleagues and the relevant clinical staff, using carefully thought-out open questions. This raises people's awareness of the issue and gives you an opportunity to hear different perspectives. Listening attentively may enable you to identify factors that could hinder change, and the information, skills and resources that staff might need in order to make the change. You may also discover who shares your views.

If appropriate, talk about any feedback you are getting from people in your classes, and about the benefits of the change to parents and to staff. In the process, you may build up a group of people who are also prepared to question an attitude, practice or procedure.

If a number of parents question the need for a certain procedure or intervention and found it unhelpful or distressing, you may need to gather further information and evidence before you take any action. Depending on the issue, your sources could include intervention rates, comparisons with other units, or a literature search. You could also approach local branches or the national offices of the relevant voluntary organizations (e.g the National Childbirth Trust, the Maternity Alliance) or The Association for Improvements in Maternity Services to ask for feedback from their members (see 'Useful addresses').

Then, you and your colleagues might:

- approach the relevant manager or person in authority to discuss the issue and present your evidence
- identify the skills and information that staff might need in order to

implement the change, and suggest ways in which these needs could be met
- write a proposal for a trial or a survey of local practices or consumer satisfaction in relation to a specific aspect of care
- raise the matter with the local Maternity Services Liaison Committee or the local branch of the Royal College of Midwives.

Key points

- Managing change is seldom easy, and requires thought and planning.
- There are several essential steps to take into account. These include:
  - finding at least one other person who supports your views
  - choosing one issue and checking that it is an appropriate time to raise it
  - gathering and evaluating the evidence for the change
  - involving people in the process
  - identifying the benefits of the change
  - identifying and reducing resistance to the change
  - offering people the skills and information they will need to effect the change.

References

Guirdham, M. (1990). *Interpersonal Skills at Work*, p. 229. Prentice Hall.

Ogden, J. (2001). From protocol to practice: who needs research? *The Lancet*, **357**, 482.

Plant, R. (1987). *Managing Change and Making it Stick*. Fontana/Collins.

And finally . . .

At the end of each antenatal course, the parents you have been working with will leave. You have given them information, passed on skills, and offered them opportunities to review their attitudes and beliefs and to discuss them with each other. Now they must handle their own individual experiences of labour, birth and parenting in their own unique ways.

You may have great hopes for them, or perhaps some fears. You probably wonder if they enjoyed the classes, or were they just being polite? Will they remember anything you have taught them? Perhaps they won't find anything useful at all. Whatever your feelings, the reality is that it is now up to the parents in whom you have invested so much. They will use or reject what you covered in your classes. They may adapt what you taught and use information and skills in ways you have not thought of. The circumstances in which they find themselves may be very different from those you envisaged. So the end of the course heralds a new beginning. Ultimately it is now up to them.

We now find ourselves in a similar position. We have spent many years focusing our attention on the needs of class leaders, and many months writing this book. We have set out our ideas and approaches, and tried to prompt reflection and reassessment. Now it is up to you.

This book is just a launching pad. Our hope is that you have found it thought provoking. There is no right way to lead antenatal classes, just as there is no one way to give birth or to parent. You are the best person to assess and respond to the needs of the people who come to your classes. You know about the circumstances in which they give birth and care for their children.

We hope you enjoy being a class leader and find it rewarding and fun.

Useful addresses

We have kept this list brief, because there are numerous organizations involved in pregnancy and childbearing, and because addresses and telephone numbers tend to change. The addresses we list here are correct at the time of publishing. They are either mentioned in the text or are key organizations, some of which hold information about a range of related organizations.

Association for Improvements in the Maternity Services (AIMS), 21 Iver Lane, Buckinghamshire SL0 9LH. Website: www.aims.org.uk. Provides information and publications on a range topics related to pregnancy and childbirth.

Disability, Pregnancy and Parenthood International. Unit F9 89/93, Fonthill Road, London N4 3JH. The national centre for disabled parents. Website: www.freespace.virgin.net/disabled.parents

Maternity Alliance, 45 Beech Street, London EC2P 2LX. Website: www.maternityalliance.org.uk. Produces a range of publications and focuses on women and families with special needs – on low incomes, with disabilities, or from minority ethnic groups.

Midwives Information and Resource Service (MIDIRS), 9 Elmdale Road, Bristol BS8 1SL. Website: www.midirs.org. Provides information on midwifery issues, a range of resources, and addresses for other relevant organizations.

Pink Parents, Website: www.pinkparents.uk.com. Provides information and support for and about gay, lesbian and bisexual parenting.

PROSPECT, 15 Park Avenue, London NW11 7SL. Website: www.schott-media/prospect. Offers training workshops for health professionals on leading antenatal classes and other topics.

SHAP Working Party on World Religions in Education, The National Society's RE Centre, 36 Causton Street, London SW1 4AU. Produces the SHAP calendar of religious festivals.

The Children's Project, Freepost SEA 10364, Richmond, Surrey TW10 7BR. Website: www.childrensproject.co.uk. Publishes and distributes *The Social Baby* and *Ethan's First Half Hour* – a series of 10 A4 photographs for use in classes.

The National Childbirth Trust (NCT), Alexandra House, Oldham Terrace, London W3 6NH. Website: www.nct-online.org. Provides information about the NCT and local contacts.

The National Childbirth Trust Maternity Sales, 239 Shawbridge Street, Glasgow G43 1QN. Website: www.nctms.co.uk. Produces a catalogue which includes books, leaflets and teaching aids.

Index